SuperJuicing

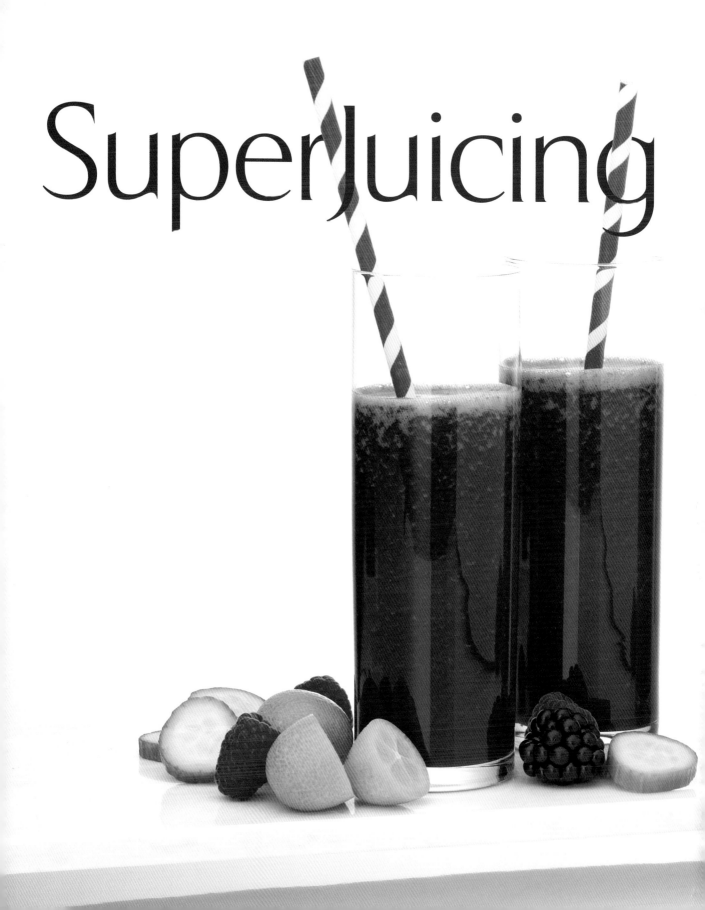

SuperJuicing

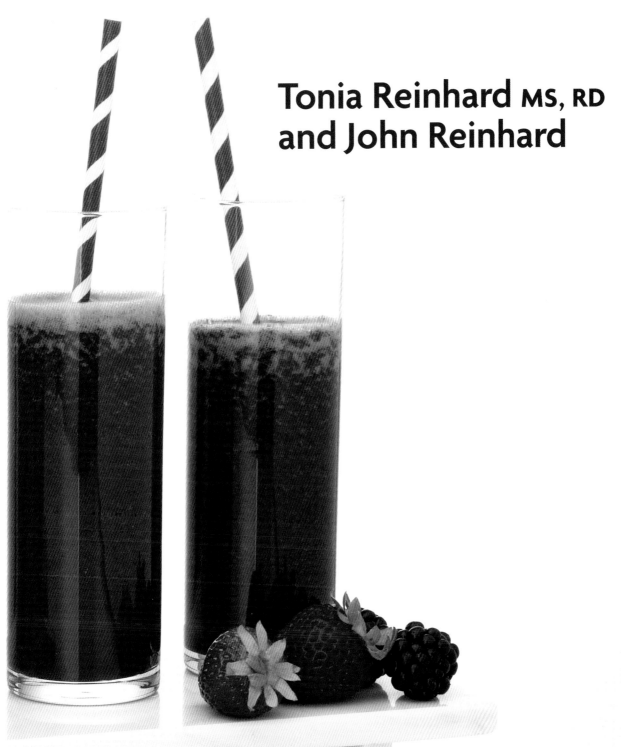

Tonia Reinhard MS, RD and John Reinhard

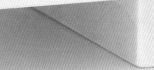

FIREFLY BOOKS

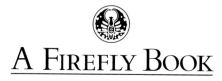

A FIREFLY BOOK

Published by Firefly Books Ltd. 2014
Copyright © 2014 Firefly Books Ltd.
Text Copyright © 2014 Tonia Reinhard
Photography Copyright © 2014 Hal Roth Photography

Second Printing

Publisher Cataloging-in-Publication Data (U.S.)
Reinhard, Tonia.
Super juicing : more than 100 nutritious vegetable and fruit recipes / Tonia Reinhard ; John Reinhard.
[240] pages : color photos ; cm.
Includes bibliographical references and index.
Summary: A comprehensive guide to using this nutrient-dense approach to eating for adults and children.
ISBN-13: 978-1-77085-307-2 (pbk.)
 1. Vegetables juices. 2. Fruit juices. 3. Smoothies (Beverages). 4. Cooking. I. Reinhard, John. II. Title.
641.3/4 dc23   TX840.J84R456   2014

Library and Archives Canada Cataloguing in Publication
A CIP record for this title is available from Library and Archives Canada

Published in the United States by
Firefly Books (U.S.) Inc.
P.O. Box 1338, Ellicott Station
Buffalo, New York 14205

Published in Canada by
Firefly Books Ltd.
50 Staples Avenue, Unit 1
Richmond Hill, Ontario L4B 0A7

Photographer: Hal Roth Photography
Food Stylist: Julie Zambonelli
Prop Stylist: Oksana Slavutych
Digital Technical Assistants: Paolo Cristante & Eric Brazier
Design and typesetting: Gareth Lind, LINDdesign
Icons: Dutch Icon and Scott Mooney

Printed in China

The publisher gratefully acknowledges the financial support for our publishing program by the Government of Canada through the Canada Book Fund as administered by the Department of Canadian Heritage.

Previous Spread:
Three-Berry Kumquat
— recipe on page 124

Acknowledgments

A hearty thanks to Brendan Reinhard for help with developing recipes and coordinating testing, and Steve and Sue Francis, owners of the Country Smokehouse in Imlay City, Michigan, for the use of their state-of-the-art test kitchen (countrysmokehouseinc.com).

Also many thanks to Faye Woodside, JD, for assistance with editing and recipe development, Zoe Violet Woodside (2 years old at the time of publication) for serving on the tasting panel and John Reinhard for his contributions to writing and research.

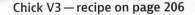

Chick V3 — recipe on page 206

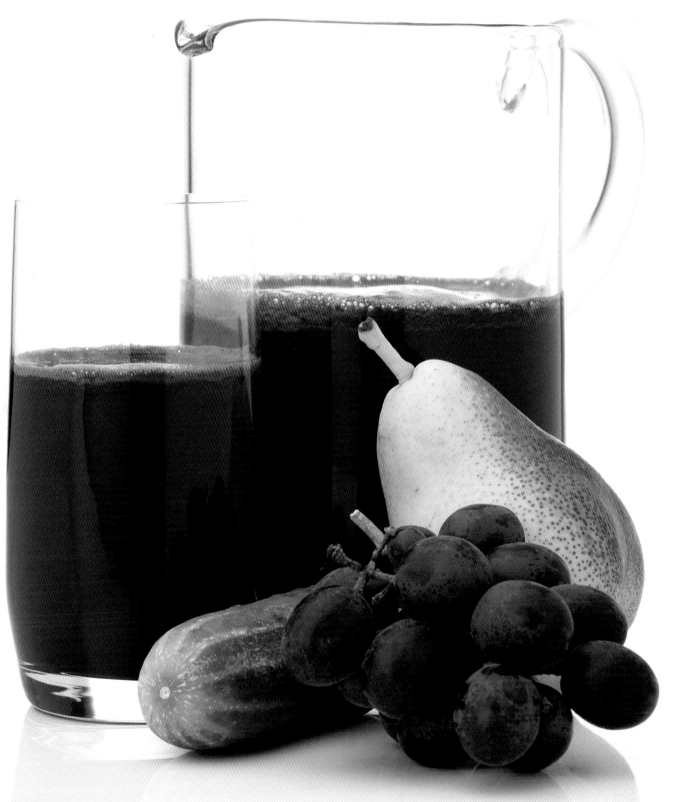

Beeted Pear on the Vine
— recipe on page 127

Contents

Gingersnap
— recipe on page 193

Preface

As a dietitian, I always steered people away from drinking high-calorie beverages. I would point out that it is more enjoyable and satisfying for most people to eat rather than drink their calories. At some point, however, I realized that, with my hectic teaching schedule, which often precluded sitting down to eat, I myself was drinking my lunch and afternoon snack. I wasn't doing any actual juicing, but I'd shake some yogurt, water, cocoa and chia seeds up in a jar and take it along with me. I'd also pack a homemade energy drink with whey protein, grapefruit juice and caffeinated diet soda for a late afternoon pick-me-up.

Not long after this revelation, I met a colleague at a local coffee shop — an awesome dietitian who's always up to date on the latest nutrition research, Aarti Batavia, owner of Nutrition & Wellness Consulting. I noticed that she too was drinking some type of home-made shake she had brought. This motivated me to find out more about real juicing, from both a health and nutrition standpoint, as well as from one that most of us can relate to: eating well in a hurry.

Although I'd been teaching at a university, working with clients and writing about nutrition for several years, it wasn't until I wrote my last book that I realized the real power of food for improving health — and, unfortunately, the power of the myths about food. In writing *Superfoods: The Healthiest Foods on the Planet*, I concentrated on reviewing the scientific studies of the nutrients and phytochemicals in foods and even studies of specific foods. The parts of the puzzle came together for me, and the central concept that emerged was one I'd learned about when I was still in school studying nutrition: nutrient density.

Nutrient density describes a cost-benefit analysis approach to eating. The idea is to consider what each food brings to the table (its complement of nutrients and phytochemicals, or lack thereof) versus how many calories we have to "give up" to eat it. It's similar to making a purchase at the store and scanning a credit card. In that transaction, we want the most and best product for our hard-earned money. We need to start thinking of our calories in much the same way. Most of us can't afford too many extra calories, considering the international statistics pointing to the planet's collective bulging waistline.

Well, nutrient density is a great concept for health and weight management, but having taught classes to moms with young children — the pickiest of eaters — it's obvious the food also has to taste good. In fact, when I teach about feeding young children, I often suggest the "stealth" model, which refers to sneaking healthy vegetables into combination foods that children will readily accept without even realizing that they just ate two servings of carrots. Juicing and blending provide an excellent camouflage for the picky eater or, as their adult counterparts may prefer to be called, the "nutrient density challenged."

Juicing and blending can also be a boon to the avid gardener. Every summer, our bountiful garden produces a surfeit of herbs and veggies, but as every backyard farmer knows, we can eat only so much steamed zucchini, roasted zucchini and zucchini bread. Basil, arugula and rosemary plants also produce huge yields but are used in relatively small quantities in most recipes. Juicing and blending provide a great way to incorporate some of these superfoods into beverages, soups, sauces and more. Not everyone has the time or space for gardening. Yet as produce prices continue to soar, a garden can be an amazingly good deal — nutrient-dense food saving you calories and money.

As you can see, juicing and blending can help you eat health-fully in a hurry (or on the run), get the most nutrient bang for your caloric buck, sneak those nutrient-dense foods into your family's diet, take your garden beyond zucchini bread — and leap tall buildings in a single bound. The last challenge, though, is to dispel the numerous myths surrounding nutrition in general and juicing in particular. In a way, dispelling the myths also requires expanding perceptions about juicing and blending, that is, looking a bit beyond the banana-strawberry smoothie. In this book, we want you to consider how various superfoods can be combined for new textures and flavors while providing a nutrition-packed and delicious beverage. We hope that this book fulfills these objectives and, most of all, that you will have fun and enjoy improving your nutritional health.

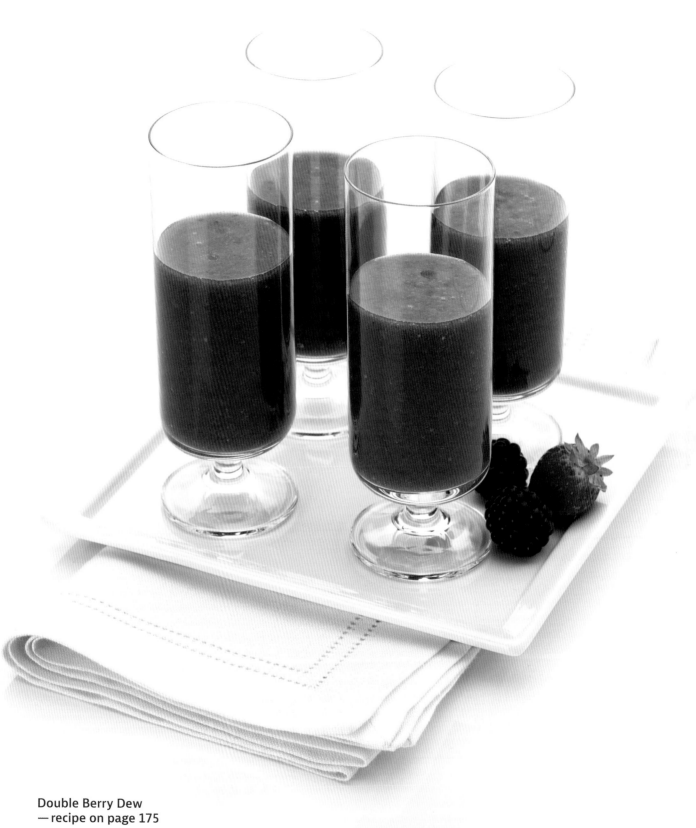

Double Berry Dew
— recipe on page 175

How To Use this Book

I F YOU'VE OPENED this book, you are most likely trying to make your diet healthier. You may be tempted to skip straight to the recipe section, which is perfectly fine, and if so, skip to Section 2. However, cultivating a healthy diet is more than just adding a few recipes that include flaxseed and blue-green algae, or whatever the superfood *du jour* happens to be. It requires changing the way you understand and think about food. For that reason, we've laid out the book in the following way: The first section of the book, "Juicing Fundamentals," includes chapters covering key points about juicing, basic nutrition principles and some general tips for making your juicing experience as fun and healthful as possible. So if you have a good handle on these topics, skip ahead to the next section. You can always come back to the first section later, or use it as a reference.

The second section contains the recipes, and the first chapter of this section includes important recipe information. Then the recipes are organized based on juicer recipes, which come first, and blender or food processor recipes. Within those two basic recipe categories, sweet beverage recipes come first, with savory or soup recipes last.

See page 90 for recipes made with a juicer, and page 148 for recipes made with a blender or food processor. Juicer recipes will yield a true juice, of thin consistency, whereas blender recipes yield thick smoothies, which preserve the fiber content of the ingredients. You'll find more information on the advantages of each method back in Chapter 1, "The Why of Juicing." The final section of the book provides you with additional resources, including a glossary and useful websites for accurate, helpful nutrition information.

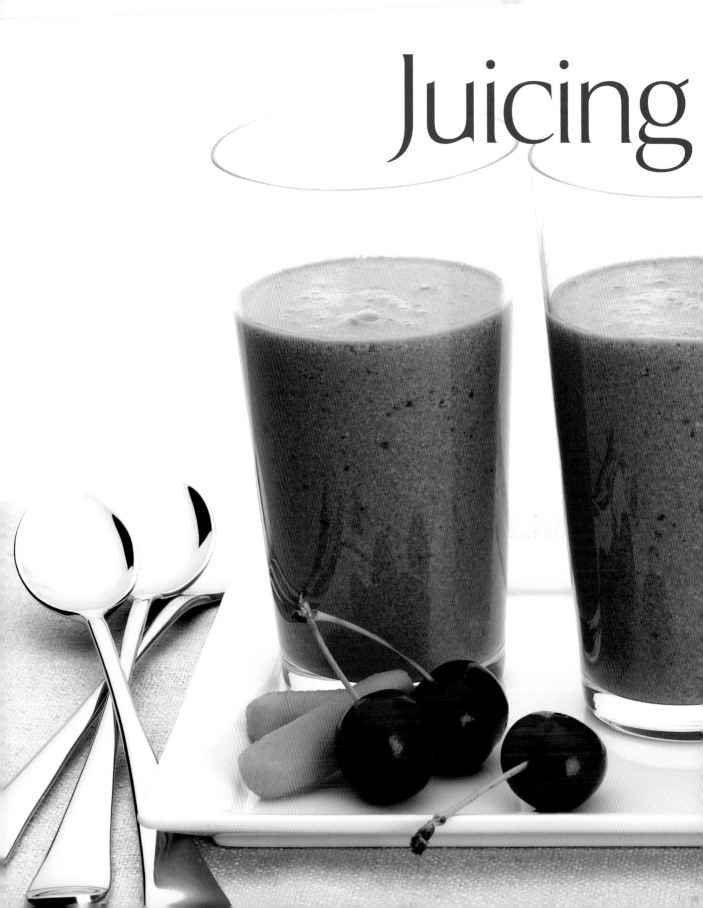

Juicing

Fundamentals

Tofu Tart — recipe on page 167

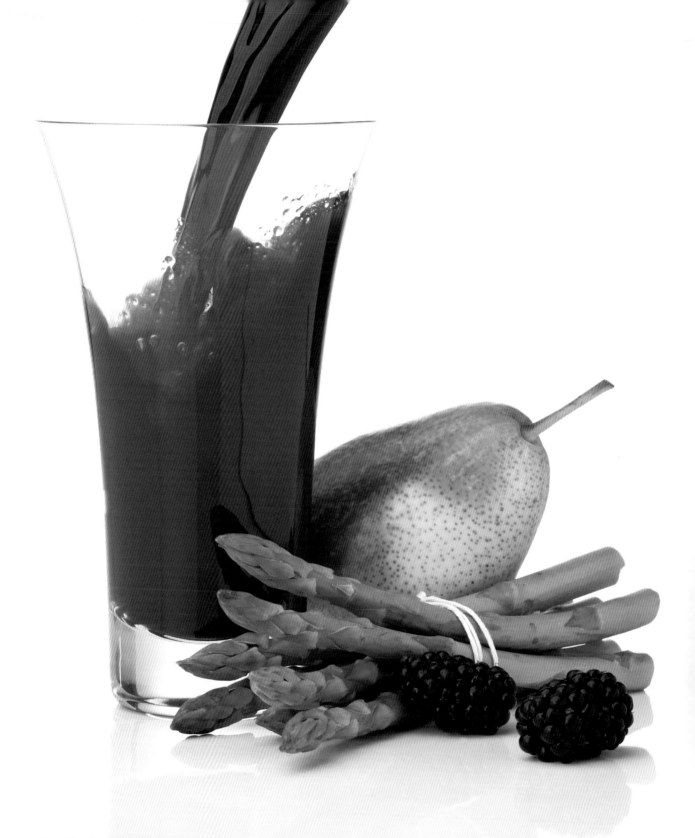

Bosc Berried Asparagus
— recipe on page 122

Chapter 1

The Why of Juicing

J UICING OFFERS MANY advantages to those who want to improve the nutritional quality of their diets, but you also need to be aware of potential pitfalls. The first order of business is to define some of the terms used in juicing and the first distinction is the difference between a juice and a smoothie. While there is no standard definition, most people consider juicing to involve a juicing machine that extracts the liquid portion from fruits and vegetables, separating it from the pulp, or fibrous component. It is generally more liquid in nature, but this varies depending on the ingredients used. A smoothie is made by using a blender or food processor. All the ingredients are added to the blender jar and the result is a thicker consistency product, since it contains some of the fibrous matter. There are advantages and disadvantages to both methods (more about that later), so this book provides recipes for both methods.

One reason to use juicing is that it allows you to prepare a highly nutritious meal replacement when you're on the move. Between work and other obligations, most of us have hectic lifestyles. We don't always have time to sit down to a breakfast or lunch that includes ample servings of fruits, vegetables and other healthy foods. More likely, we might be tempted by the promise of fast and tasty food at the local drive-through. If, instead, we take a few minutes before we leave the house to prepare a healthy and well-balanced mix of superfoods and ensure that it's packaged safely, we'll have a great-tasting and healthy meal at the ready.

Another advantage to juicing is that some people don't like the taste of many vegetables, particularly those at the higher nutrient end, for example superfoods like kale. But they do like fruit, and the vegetables can be combined with the fruit for added nutrients without adversely affecting the taste. In light of the current recommendations to increase fruit and vegetable intake, it's important for those who are not avid veggie eaters to find other ways to incorporate these health-promoting foods into their diet.

A related benefit of juicing is the ability to use superfood ingredients that may not necessarily lend themselves to more straightforward consumption. Take blue-green algae as an example: Most of us don't want to sit down to a bowl of this superfood and spoon it in. However, it's a nutrient-dense food packed with vitamin C, B vitamins and more. In fact, a mere ¼ of a teaspoon (1 mL) contains an entire day's supply of vitamin B12, a nutrient in which national surveys indicate that up to 15% of those over the age of 51 may be deficient (the percentage is even higher in vegetarians). Adding a teaspoon (5 mL) to a tasty smoothie is an easy and palatable way to incorporate this superfood into one's diet.

For those with children, juicing is a great way to introduce them to new fruits and vegetables and let them participate. Studies have shown that when children participate in food and meal preparation, they are more accepting of the foods. It's probably easy to see, in the case of juicing, that not only will children be more interested in tasting the juice product that they help make, but also the whole fruits and vegetables that went into the juice. This probably applies more to an older child, but juicing can also be a way to circumvent the perennial eating problem in younger children, that of the picky eater who refuses to eat any type of vegetable. Juicing provides a stealthy way to include healthy vegetables into both meals and stand-alone juices or smoothies. For example, a healthy blend of carrots and winter squash will not be detected in spaghetti sauce or chili.

The Advantages of Juicing: Setting the Record Straight

You can see that there are plenty of reasons to do juicing, enough that we don't need to fall back on the myths of juicing, which include mistaken concepts such as raw foods diets, enzymes, cleansing and detoxification. But let's take a look at one of the most common myths: A food's enzymes need to be released and consumed intact. This myth begins with the idea that nutrients are "trapped" in some portion of the whole food, typically the plant wall, which is made up of dietary fiber in the form of cellulose.

A careful examination of the science gives us the reason why this is not accurate: The cell wall of plant foods is easily disrupted both in the chewing process and in various food preparation processes and cooking. In other words, your teeth do plenty of damage to plant walls without recourse to a 2,000 rpm juice machine engine. Now, it's possible (and in fact more likely) that plant matter such as cellulose will bind to nutrients inside the gastrointestinal tract to prevent absorption of the nutrient. This most commonly occurs with essential minerals, such as iron and zinc.

Before you use this absorption issue to justify becoming a meata-tarian, remember that cellulose is a form of dietary fiber. Based on all the studies to date, most people don't consume enough fiber. There are many reasons why a person might become deficient in essential minerals, especially iron, but given dietary intake studies, fiber consumption is not one of them. Dietary fiber has been shown to promote health, help prevent a variety of chronic diseases and potentially aid in weight loss (more on dietary fiber in Chapter 2 "Nutrition and Health Basics").

The next part of the myth purports that the enzymes present in foods are somehow biologically active, or active inside the body. It's true that foods contain enzymes. Pineapple and papaya, for example, contain the enzymes bromelain and papain, respectively, which are used in commercial tenderizers to break down muscle fibers in meat. If pineapple enzymes break down muscle fibers, how come pina coladas turn your brain to figurative but not literal mush? The answer lies in the fact that enzymes, whether from food or from the human body itself, are proteins.

Here's how it works: One of the first steps in the process of digesting the food we eat is that the stomach releases strong acids and some digestive enzymes. The acid changes the protein in the food, uncoiling its spring-like shape, a process known as denaturation. Other common ways to denature a protein include agitation and applying heat. You do this every time you cook an egg, of which the egg white is pure protein. After cracking the egg into a hot pan, you'll notice that the egg white soon changes from clear and liquid to solid and white. When you make meringue by beating egg whites at high speed, the egg whites undergo the same process, that of denaturation.

While these may be tasty examples of food science in the kitchen, denaturation is a job-changer for the protein, which now loses its functionality. In digestion, uncoiling, or denaturing, proteins is an important step in providing the human digestive enzymes to penetrate these large proteins and break them down into their constituent parts, amino acids. So you can see that by the time an enzyme in a food, like papaya's papain, goes from the stomach to the small intestine, it will be broken down into its constituent parts and won't be able to do whatever job or function it had.

What about the myth that eating foods in their raw state is essential for obtaining all the nutrients and deriving special benefits from the food? The first part of this myth we must unpack is the notion that foods contain a "life force" beyond what scientists are able to identify or measure in chemical analysis of the food. If there were such a compound or force, it's most likely that it would've been detected by now. The next part is less straightforward and presents the idea that cooking destroys nutrients.

This is accurate for some nutrients, but just the opposite for others. Some nutrients (more on this in Chapter 2, "Nutrition and Health Basics") are sensitive to heat and are lost in prolonged cooking times. One example is the B vitamin folate, or in supplement form, folic acid. Folate also evaporates readily into the atmosphere, so a significant amount will be lost by just storing foods containing it, such as leafy greens, for too long in the refrigerator.

In the case of other nutrients, however, some are better absorbed once the foods that contain them have been cooked. An example of this is any of the carotenoids, a large group of compounds that are powerful antioxidants. The carotenoid lycopene has been widely touted as protective against certain cancers, especially prostate cancer. Tomatoes are an excellent source of lycopene, but it is best absorbed and used by the body when it has been heated for a long period, which is why highly processed foods containing tomato sauce and paste, such as spaghetti sauce, ketchup and pizza sauce, are far better sources of lycopene than the raw tomatoes used to make them. In fact, epidemiologic studies show that men who consume higher amounts of these foods have lower rates of prostate cancer.

The answer seems to be, then, to make sure your diet intake contains a mix of foods that are raw, which is also good for the teeth by stimulating bone growth and maintaining healthy gums, and those that you cook.

How about the related myths of detoxification and cleansing? First we need to challenge the concept that the body requires cleansing and detoxification that it can't perform on its own. The average person consumes a half-ton (450 kg) of food and beverages every year.

The human gastrointestinal tract is ideally suited to consume foods, break them down to the smallest components, absorb what is needed and excrete what is not. Most of this happens in the roughly 28 feet (8.5 m) of the small intestine, which, if laid out flat, has an absorptive surface roughly the size of a tennis court. The large intestine handles the waste by moving it along its length and reabsorbing water and electrolytes and allowing microbes to act on the waste. It's hard to imagine that, given this level of sophistication and precision, the system is deficient to the extent of requiring assistance from us in completing these tasks.

That being said, the evidence is clear that eating certain foods — or juicing and drinking them, for that matter — can help the work of the intestine along. Moving waste out of the body quickly and efficiently could arguably be called "detoxifying," but it isn't the result of a special recipe or mystical berry. It's the normal effect of dietary fiber (more on dietary fiber in Chapter 2, "Nutrients and Health Basics"). Dietary fiber has two primary beneficial effects on intestinal function. First, it adds bulk to the stool, which promotes movement through the gastrointestinal tract and quicker elimination. This leaves less time for any hypothetical toxins that are present in the waste to do any damage. Second, fiber turns into compounds called short-chain fatty

Did You Know?

The average person consumes a half-ton (450 kg) of food and beverages every year.

acids that can neutralize toxins. Here's how it works: Bacteria in the colon consume the fiber and release the fatty acids. More fatty acids mean a higher level of acid in the colon. The higher level of acid prevents a normal process whereby the body turns generally inoffensive compounds into toxic or carcinogenic compounds. The fatty acids also feed other bacteria, which in turn metabolize toxic compounds, making them harmless.

Jumping Over the Juicing Pitfalls

While the benefits of juicing are evident, it's important to be aware of and avoid a few potential pitfalls. First and foremost is to understand that when juicing or making smoothies, you are condensing calorie-containing foods into a small volume. For example, a normal-size grapefruit, about the size of a softball, is about 100 calories. After placing it in a blender, the yield is about 10 fluid ounces (300 mL). It takes the average person much longer to eat a grapefruit than swallow a glass of juice. If not attentive to the calories in juices, you could easily gain weight.

Another problem for some people is that they don't feel as satisfied when drinking caloric beverages compared to eating an equivalent number of calories. The feeling of being satisfied in relation to eating foods is known as satiety. So a person for whom drinking a juice or smoothie doesn't result in the same level of satiety as eating solid foods may drink the beverage then eat additional solids to feel satiated. For this reason, it's important to think of juices and smoothies as a part of the total diet, in that one of these drinks replaces the equivalent number of calories from a food.

While this satiety issue is not true for all people, it is important to be aware that it could be true for you. In fact, some studies have shown that replacing meals with drinks can help some people lose weight. This is a case of knowing yourself and what works best for you. If you think you are one of the people not satisfied with drinking their calories, consider adding some of the super enhancers or other ingredients that studies have shown may help either increase satiety or promote weight loss in other ways. But remember to carefully consider the total calories and use the juices or smoothies more as meal replacements.

Juice or Smoothie?

Both methods present advantages and disadvantages, and, in all instances, one method's advantage represents a disadvantage of the other method!

Let's start with the positive. The first advantage to using a blender or food processor is that most people have one and will not have to purchase another kitchen appliance. Another advantage, and this one is probably the most important, is that in blending the ingredients and not producing a pulp, which is characteristic of the juicing process, you obtain all the dietary fiber from the ingredients. With juicing, the liquid portion of the ingredients, or the juice, is extracted from the whole food, leaving behind all the fibrous components. If you save the pulp and incorporate it into other recipes, you can save the dietary fiber for a later date. And indeed some of the recipes (All Things Pulp, page 147, Peaches 'n' Cream Oatmeal, page 144, and Peppered Pasta, page 146) show you how to do just that, but it is an additional step in the process, which many people will not be inclined to do.

The main advantage of the juicing process is that you don't have to highly process the ingredients before using them because the juicer does it for you. For example, you can place an intact pineapple in the juicer instead of having to perform the laborious task of removing the skin and core. This is obviously not the case with a blender, in which you must remove certain nonedible components before processing and, depending on the item, this may take a significant amount of time. The other major advantage to the juicer is that some people may prefer the consistency, which is more fluid, while the blender makes a thicker consistency. As mentioned, we have recipes for both methods, and more information is coming in Chapter 5, "The How-To of Juicing."

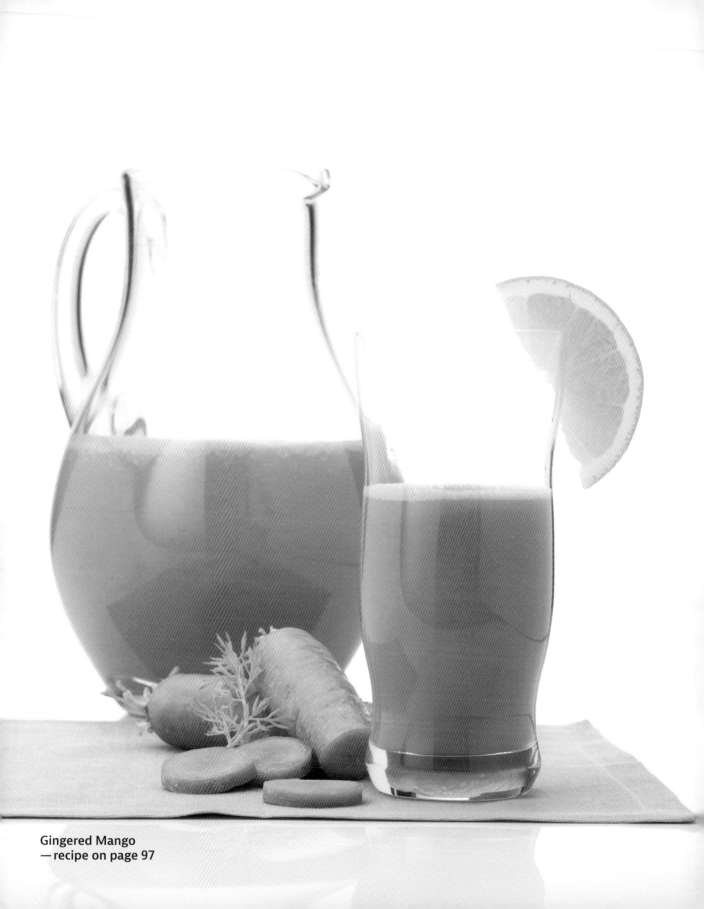

Gingered Mango
— recipe on page 97

Chapter 2

Nutrition and Health Basics

MOST PEOPLE eat without thinking too much about what's in their food, and most of us eat and drink up to a half-ton (450 kg) of foods and beverages every year! Some people are just naturally interested in nutrition and health and want to know more about the connection. For others, it may take a new health concern, such as being told by their physician that their cholesterol is too high, to start learning more about the foods they eat. Either way, one thing is clear: The nutrition we obtain from the foods we eat can either promote health and longer life expectancy, or it can work against good health. In the recipe section of the book, you'll see the nutritional highlights of each entry, so this background section on nutrition and health can be a valuable reference for understanding what each nutrient does to promote health and fight disease.

Let's Dig Deeper

In much the same way that scientists learned that material objects were made up of smaller parts, namely molecules and atoms, so we have found that the foods we eat are made up of nutrients, some of which are simple elements while others are complex molecules. Looking at a food label for bread, we'd find ingredients like flour and oil, but we can dig deeper to find out what's in the flour. So let's take a closer look at what exactly is in our food.

The body needs six groups or types of nutrients, often called essential, which means we need these compounds to survive and our body can't make them, or can't make them in sufficient amounts, although we'll see that the definition of essential gets stretched for some nutrients. The six groups are water, carbohydrate, protein, fat (or lipids), vitamins and minerals.

Start with the Essentials

Did You Know?

The body needs six groups or types of nutrients, often called essential, which means we need these compounds to survive and our body can't make them, or can't make them in sufficient amounts.

Everyone has heard the adage "You are what you eat." This couldn't be more accurate when considering what nutrition is all about. It's not a flattering comparison, but the human body contains the same proportion of the essential nutrients as an ear of corn. This unflattering analogy shows that the human body is made up of similar compounds as the foods we eat, which is why they provide us with nutrition. Basically, we eat food containing thousands of compounds and our digestive system breaks the food down to its smallest parts and then uses the essential nutrients to build and repair cells and tissues. As mentioned, the word "essential" refers to the need to obtain these compounds through our foods, since our body can't make them. Adults don't grow as do infants and children, except, unfortunately, in a horizontal direction, but the adult body needs to repair and replace body tissues.

The adult body contains an estimated 50 trillion to 100 trillion cells, not all of which can be replaced but many of which must be replaced on a routine basis. As an example, the red blood cell, which carries oxygen throughout the body, has a life span of about four months. So the body is continually in the business of replacing old cells, and interestingly, the body recycles many of its components: Red blood cells go green! To make new red blood cells, the body needs specific nutrients in certain amounts — building blocks for all forms of life.

Our new red blood cell will need nutrients from each of the six essential nutrient groups: water, carbohydrate, fat, protein, minerals and vitamins. From each group, this particular cell will need several specific nutrients, which might be slightly different from what is needed for other cells. While we need all the essential nutrients, we need some on an immediate basis to continue living, and of these, water is the most crucial in the short term. We can survive for quite some time without replenishing our stores of vitamin D, but we would die within days if short on water. This applies to all the nutrients, so a deficiency of some nutrients will cause a problem sooner than a deficiency of others.

Another type of nutrient that is critical in the short term is energy. Of the six groups, only fat, carbohydrate and protein provide energy in the form of calories. For each of the trillions of cells, water and energy will be the most crucial nutrients needed within days.

While each essential nutrient has a specific job that no other nutrient can do, three groups — water, vitamins and minerals — help the body obtain energy from the other three groups: carbohydrate, fat and protein. Most people know they need energy to perform physical activity, but they may not know that the body also needs energy to build and repair its parts — blood, bone and muscle. The body is a sort of walking chemistry lab performing hundreds of millions of chemistry experiments, or reactions, every day of our lives. And to extend the metaphor, the vitamins, of the group of six, are the busy chemists working overtime to turn the food we eat into the building materials we need for repair.

A Bit about Each Group

Water

Most of us don't think of water as an essential nutrient alongside vitamins and other more familiar nutrients. It's so essential to life, however, that when we're deprived of it, even for a short time, we die. That being said, the myths surrounding water intake abound, so let's tackle them.

From a chemical standpoint, water is simplicity itself, containing two hydrogen atoms and one oxygen atom. It is this simple form that accounts for all of water's functions, the most important being its role

Did You Know?

While each essential nutrient has a specific job that no other nutrient can do, three groups — water, vitamins and minerals — help the body obtain energy from the other three groups: carbohydrate, fat and protein.

as the perfect solvent and medium for chemical reactions in the body.

Another of water's functions is that it brings nutrients to each cell and carries away waste products from the cell to be excreted from the body. In addition, water is the main constituent of every cell and the tissues and organs that the cells make up. It lubricates the gastrointestinal tract and other body tissues, as well as cushioning joints. Water is critical to help regulate body temperature because of its capacity to change temperature slowly.

So how much water do we need? It all depends on body size, caloric intake and any special conditions, such as engaging in strenuous physical activity, particularly in a hot or humid climate, or taking prescription medications called diuretics. Without these conditions, the average person needs 1 milliliter of water for every calorie they eat. A person's age also influences the need for fluid, with infants requiring a higher proportion because their body composition includes a higher amount of water. A typical woman, standing 5 foot 5 (165 cm) and weighing 125 pounds (57 kg), should consume about 2,000 calories. Her daily need for water is 2,000 milliliters, or 2 liters (2 quarts). But here's where two major myths come in: She does not need to drink 2 liters every day, and she does not need to drink this fluid as water.

We get about half the water we need from the food we eat, and we get the water we need from any fluid we drink. Foods consist of anywhere from 50% to 90% water, with some foods, such as fruits and vegetables, at the higher end of the range. People who eat lots of fruits and vegetables get more water than a meat and potatoes eater. Any beverage we drink provides mostly water. The main benefit from drinking plain water is that it hydrates and does not provide calories.

Oh, and one last myth is that caffeinated beverages do not provide fluid. Studies have proven that coffee and tea, although they promote urination, still provide fluid, or water.

In many ways, juicing is a perfect way to stay hydrated, since it provides not only the water we need, but other essential nutrients as a bonus.

Carbohydrates

This group of nutrients has been taking it on the chin ever since Dr. Atkins convinced millions of people to buy bacon and forgo the fruit. While he had some good points about the adverse effects of a diet too high in carbohydrate, the latest research suggests it's all about the types of carbohydrates in the diet, not so much the amount.

As a class of compounds, the main function of carbohydrate is to serve as the body's preferred source of energy. One important distinction among the different types is whether the carbohydrate is a complex carbohydrate or a simple carbohydrate. And even within that distinction, most foods contain a mix, so the important consideration is which form, complex or simple, is present in the highest amount.

Simple carbohydrates are primarily the sugars in our foods, and the most common form is glucose. Glucose is the main form of energy used by the body's cells, and it travels in our blood to all the cells providing fuel. This is reflected in a lab value you may have had your physician comment on, your blood glucose level. It's important that it stay within a specific range, because if it's too low, the body's cells begin to starve, and when it's too high, as in diabetes, it damages blood vessels and body tissues.

Complex carbohydrate consists of starch and fiber. The body digests starch and produces energy. In contrast, humans don't have the enzymes to break down fiber, so it does not provide significant energy. However, it serves other important functions, such as promoting regular bowel function and helping to maintain blood glucose and cholesterol levels in healthy ranges. In addition, friendly bacteria that live in the colon can use fiber for energy. When they degrade fiber, this generates other compounds that appear to improve bowel function and protect against diseases, such as cancer. Feeding these friendly bacteria is important, because researchers are continually finding more ways these bacteria promote health and prevent a variety of diseases, not just those affecting the gut. They have discovered that these bacteria, or our gut microbiome, which consist of about 40 species and number in the trillions, are as distinctive to a person as a fingerprint.

One of the reasons why fiber helps maintain regular bowel function is that it acts like a sponge to attract water to help move everything along. In addition, in this sponge-like role, it can help you feel fuller after eating, which is called satiety. Studies have shown that a higher fiber intake is associated with lower body weight. Another benefit of complex carbohydrates is that the foods containing them, such as whole grains, are excellent sources of several vitamins and minerals.

As with all foods and nutrients, the best approach is essentially a balancing act. As to the amount, it depends on a person's age, gender, body weight and personal preferences. In a healthy and well-balanced diet, carbohydrate contributes about half of the total calories. If you focus on the complex carbohydrates with fiber, such as whole grains, legumes and vegetables, you'll probably get the amount your body needs. Most fruits contain simple carbohydrate — naturally occurring sugar — but nutritionally speaking, eating (or drinking) fruit is quite different from consuming other foods containing sugar. This latter group, so-called sweet treats, such as soda, sweetened drinks, candy and cookies, provide calories and sugar but, in some cases, no nutrients in return. In contrast, fruits provide fiber, vitamins and minerals.

People with diabetes or prediabetes should be planning their meals and snacks around the concept of carb counting. This is not to suggest that carbohydrate is unhealthy, but in the process of deriving energy from carbohydrate, the body produces glucose. In diabetes, the body cannot effectively handle glucose, so it rises in the blood, leading to damage that raises the risk for many other diseases, some life-threatening. By counting the carbs, a person with these conditions is more consistent in the amount and type of carbohydrate they eat and can more effectively maintain their blood glucose in a healthy range.

Fat

And yet another nutrient that has been much maligned over the years. As a group, fats play many key roles, and specific parts of dietary fats, called fatty acids, are both essential nutrients and powerful agents in fighting disease. The foods we eat provide fat, the body stores energy as fat and, in both cases, these are triglycerides. When it comes to storing fat, which not many of us like to do, if we had to store our energy reserves as carbohydrate, we'd be huge! Fat takes up about half the space, in chemical terms, as carbohydrate. So we can see that fat is the perfect form of storing extra energy in the body, and it's also the reason that fat has a higher calorie value: 9 calories per gram, compared to carbohydrate and protein at 4 calories per gram.

Another key function of fat is to insulate the body against temperature extremes. This same insulation function also protects the organs by cushioning them. On the micro scale, fats connect together to make up the protective membranes surrounding each body cell and other critical structures. As anyone who has tried a very low-fat diet knows, fat in foods adds to flavor, texture and "mouth feel," the technical term that describes the creamy sensation in your mouth when you eat a food containing fat, such as ice cream. Another aspect of dietary fat you may have noticed on a low-fat diet is that fat contributes to satiety, which is why you were probably hungrier on that low-fat diet.

And now for the nutritional punches from fat: We need fat to be able to absorb vitamins that are dissolvable in fat, known as fat-soluble vitamins. These include vitamins A, D, E and K. This is a problem for people with diseases that mean the body cannot absorb fat, since they will not absorb these essential vitamins. More recently, scientists have studied numerous compounds in plants called phytochemicals, such as lycopene, many of which help prevent chronic diseases. Several of these important phytochemicals are also fat soluble, so without adequate dietary fat, the body will not fully absorb these protective compounds.

Certain fatty acids, the smaller compounds that form triglycerides, are essential for life, and these include linoleic and linolenic acids, found in plant oils. You may have heard about the health benefits of the Mediterranean diet. This style of eating is characterized by a higher fat intake, sometimes up to 40% of calories, rather than the typical 30% recommended by most health agencies. However, the main form of fat in this diet is polyunsaturated fat, found in fish (omega-3 fatty acids) and plants such as flax and chia seeds and walnuts, and monounsaturated fat, found in several plant oils but especially in olive oil. Many studies attest to the benefits, ranging from protection against heart disease and diabetes to various types of cancer, of including these foods in your daily diet.

Protein

Protein is the last of the trio of energy-yielding essential nutrients, but certainly not least in importance! From time to time this nutrient garners much attention as being important for bodybuilders and those trying to lose weight. Most of us get plenty of protein if we're consuming animal products of any type, although for uninformed vegetarians, and especially vegans, who use no animal products, protein could be in short supply. Of all the essential nutrients, proteins — and specifically the smaller constituents of proteins, the amino acids — truly are the building blocks of the body. To make cells, tissues and important compounds such as enzymes and antibodies, the body uses proteins. The body can make some amino acids, but nine are essential, which means the body can't make them and we must obtain them from the diet. In fact, when scientists assess the quality of a protein, one method is to consider the content of these nine essential amino acids. Foods that provide protein contain a mix of the various amino acids, both essential and nonessential.

Unlike fat, we don't have reserves or stores of protein. In the body, all protein is considered functional because it performs some type of function. The protein in muscle, for example, is structural and allows us to perform physical work. The protein in bone, hair tendons and other components also helps maintain structure. Another important way protein works is as the base for key compounds. One such group is the enzymes, which nudge chemical reactions to take place, whether it's to digest food or promote the formation of new cells. Antibodies are important components of the immune system to protect us against invaders, such as viruses and bacteria. Another major role of proteins is to serve as carrier molecules, sort of like taxis, to transport other compounds, such as vitamins, around the body where needed.

Since protein is so important, how do we know we're getting enough? Well, most people in more economically developed countries consume up to twice as much as their body needs! But there are exceptions. As mentioned, vegetarians, and especially vegans, need to be attentive to not just the amount but also the quality of the protein. In general, animal proteins are considered higher-quality and complete, which means they contain all the essential amino acids. The protein

Avocadowow
— recipe on page 204

Table 1: Fat-Soluble Vitamins

Fat-Soluble Vitamins	Function
Vitamin A	Maintain integrity of cornea, epithelial cells and mucus membranes; aid growth of skin, bone and teeth; regulate synthesis of reproductive hormones; protect immune system; protect against cancer
Vitamin D	Maintain bone tissue by regulating the absorption and excretion of calcium and phosphorus
Vitamin E	Maintain cell membranes; act as an antioxidant in fighting disease-causing free radicals and in protecting other important compounds from oxidation
Vitamin K	Regulate synthesis of blood clotting compounds; regulate calcium levels in blood

Table 2: Water-Soluble Vitamins

Water-Soluble Vitamins	Function
Vitamin C	Aid collagen synthesis; act as antioxidant; regulate immune function; enhance iron absorption; regulate synthesis of thyroid hormone; aid protein metabolism
Vitamin B1 (thiamine)	Coenzyme in energy metabolism; maintain appetite and nervous system function
Vitamin B2 (riboflavin)	Coenzyme in energy metabolism; maintain skin and visual function
Vitamin B3 (niacin)	Coenzyme in energy metabolism; maintain skin and nervous and digestive systems
Pantothenic acid	Coenzyme in energy metabolism
Biotin	Coenzyme in energy metabolism; regulate synthesis of fat and glycogen
Vitamin B6 (pyridoxine)	Coenzyme in protein and fat metabolism; regulate synthesis of red blood cells and niacin
Vitamin B12	Aid cellular synthesis; maintain nervous system function
Folate (folic acid)	Coenzyme in cellular synthesis

in plant foods tends to be of lower quality, or incomplete, in that it is missing one or more of the essential amino acids.

Another group of people who may need to increase protein are the elderly. Several studies have shown a higher-protein diet can help preserve muscle in older people as they age. People who have lost weight due to illness may also need to increase their protein intake until they regain the weight they lost. For the average person, the recommended amount of daily protein intake is based on their weight, about 36.4% of body weight. A moderately active woman weighing 115 pounds (52 kg) needs 42 grams of protein daily. With some forms of kidney disease, a person will actually need to be careful not to eat too much protein because the kidneys have difficulty excreting the byproducts of protein digestion.

Vitamins

When most people think about nutrition, the first thing that comes to mind is the vitamins. These compounds continue to be the stars of the nutrition world, and it was their discovery, in rapid succession, that fueled the explosion of research into nutrition and health. Currently, the list of vitamins known to be essential for human life is at 13 (see Tables 1 and 2), but as researchers continue to study these intriguing nutrients and other compounds in food, the list may grow.

Researchers are studying everything from how the body absorbs vitamins from different foods to how they may be involved in preventing chronic diseases. For example, even vitamin D, a long-established vitamin, is now being considered in the prevention of diseases such as diabetes, heart disease and multiple sclerosis, although before this latest research, it was mostly noted for its role in bone development and enhancement of calcium absorption.

As this exciting research into possible roles in chronic disease continues, we know the general roles these nutrients play in maintaining health. Some act like hormones — chemical messengers — in the body. Indeed, vitamin D is actually a hormone by the scientific definition. Several others are a part of enzymes, helping to control metabolic reactions in the body. It is the case for many of the enzymes with which the vitamins team up that they could not function without their vitamin partner, called coenzymes. Most of the B vitamins, for example, are coenzymes in the process of deriving energy from the food we eat.

Vitamins fall into one of two groups, those that dissolve in fat, termed fat soluble (see Table 1), and those that dissolve in water, or water soluble (see Table 2). This is a useful distinction because it tells you how a particular vitamin works in the body, how it's handled by the body and how readily it's lost from foods containing it in storage, food processing and preparation. Another important aspect of solubility related to how the body stores a vitamin tells you how easily it is lost from the body, and therefore how often it needs to consumed. This also provides an idea of how likely the vitamin is to be toxic, in that if the body stores it for a long period of time, excesses could be harmful.

In general, the body does not store water-soluble vitamins, so we need to consume them on a regular basis. They are also readily excreted by the kidneys, which means that when you consume more than you need, the excess ends up in the urine. You may have heard that taking vitamin supplements produces expensive urine, and this is somewhat accurate. It may seem wasteful, but it helps ensure that you won't store up toxic levels. When it comes to fat-soluble vitamins, however, the body does store these, and in the event of an excess, they won't be easily excreted. For this reason, fat-soluble vitamin supplements need to be carefully considered because, depending on the vitamin, it can prove fatal.

Some people think they need large quantities of vitamins, but the truth is that our need for each vitamin is extremely tiny: Adding up all the vitamins, we need about an ounce (28 g) each day. In scientific units, the amount for each vitamin varies from milligrams to just micrograms. For a sense of how little a microgram is, one microgram is one-millionth of a gram, and a gram is about one-thirtieth of an ounce! The units for other vitamins, such as vitamin A, are either retinol equivalents (RE) or international units (IU), the latter of which is used in the supplement industry for vitamins A and E.

Fruits and vegetables tend to be excellent sources of many key vitamins, especially those for which many people have inadequate intakes, such as vitamins C and A. Since this book emphasizes superfoods, or nutrient-dense foods, the recipes reflect combinations of ingredients to maximize vitamin intake. In addition, many of the disease-fighting phytochemicals (more on these later) are also present in high amounts in both the main recipe ingredients and the special added ingredients, the super enhancers.

Table 3: Major Minerals

Mineral	Function
Calcium	Aid bone and teeth formation, blood clotting, nerve transmission, muscle contraction; regulate blood pressure
Chloride	Maintain fluid balance; component of digestive juices
Magnesium	Aid muscle contraction; component of enzymes; aid energy production and transport; regulate protein production
Phosphorus	Aid bone and teeth formation; regulate metabolism of carbohydrate, fat and protein; aid ATP (energy compound) formation, kidney function, muscle contraction, nerve signaling
Potassium	Maintain the balance of water and the electrolytes, which maintains the integrity of the cells; sustain the heartbeat; may be involved with blood pressure regulation
Sodium	Maintain fluid balance outside of cells; regulate acid-base balance; influence muscle contraction; transport compounds across the cell membrane
Sulfur	Concentrated in cartilage, skin and hair and is part of thiamin and two essential amino acids, methionine and cysteine; help maintain fluid balance

Minerals

Diamonds may be forever, but so are the essential minerals that our bodies need. Long after a human body has decomposed, the minerals in our bodies remain unchanged. On the plus side of the ledger, this indestructible nature means that cooking temperatures and other types of processing food do not reduce the amounts of these nutrients in foods. One caveat, though, is that minerals are water soluble and prolonged contact with water leeches them out of foods.

Unlike the other essential nutrients, which tend to be complex molecules, minerals are the basic chemical elements familiar to us in everyday items other than food, like copper pipes and iron railings. And, as with vitamins, minerals fall into two major categories, in this case either macrominerals (also called major minerals) or trace minerals (see Tables 3 and 4). But unlike the vitamins, for which the distinction is solubility, the difference between them is in the amount we need. Macrominerals are those that the body contains in amounts greater than 5 grams, and trace minerals are present in the body in amounts less than 5 grams. This distinction is also helpful in knowing the amounts you need to consume every day. Magnesium, for example, is a macromineral, and a young adult male needs 400 milligrams each

Table 4: Trace Minerals

Mineral	Function
Chromium	Works with insulin to allow glucose to enter cells for energy or storage
Copper	Part of enzymes needed for iron metabolism; defend against free radicals; aid keratin and connective tissue formation
Fluoride	Part of fluoroapatite in bones and teeth, which hardens tooth enamel and makes bone structure more stable
Iodine	Part of thyroxine and other compounds released by the thyroid gland that regulate cellular energy and other important functions
Iron	Part of hemoglobin in blood and myoglobin in muscle carrying oxygen; involved in several enzymes that are important in energy metabolism
Manganese	Part of several enzymes, including one that fights free radicals
Molybdenum	Part of several enzymes
Selenium	Part of several enzymes, including one that fights a specific oxygen radical, that protect cell membranes from oxidative damage
Zinc	Part of more than 70 enzymes controlling vital functions, including the maintenance of acid-base balance, excretion of toxic ammonia, production of hydrochloric acid needed for digestion, protein digestion, detoxification of alcohol and formation of collagen in wound healing; critical in reproduction, growth and sexual development; crucial to appetite by affecting the senses of taste and smell

day. In contrast, he will need only 8 milligrams of iron, a trace mineral, in his daily diet. You can see that the magnitude of difference is high — about 50 times more magnesium is needed every day compared to iron.

The various essential minerals function in many different ways. Some help to maintain fluid balance and proper acidity levels, while some are involved in muscle contraction. Several minerals have more than one function. One example is calcium, which is a major constituent of bone and as such is necessary for strong skeletal tissue. In addition, calcium plays a key role in blood clotting, blood pressure regulation and muscle contraction.

As mentioned, the amount we need of each essential mineral varies depending on whether it is a macro- or trace mineral. Several minerals are inadequate in the diets of many people, for example calcium and iron. But another concern is toxicity, as many minerals are fatal in excess amounts. One such mineral is copper, which because of its potential toxicity was used years ago by the populace of Mumbai, India, as the drug of choice to commit suicide. The toxic nature of some minerals relates to how the body metabolizes them, with some being excreted when in excess, while others, such as iron, accumulate in the liver, ultimately causing liver disease and finally death.

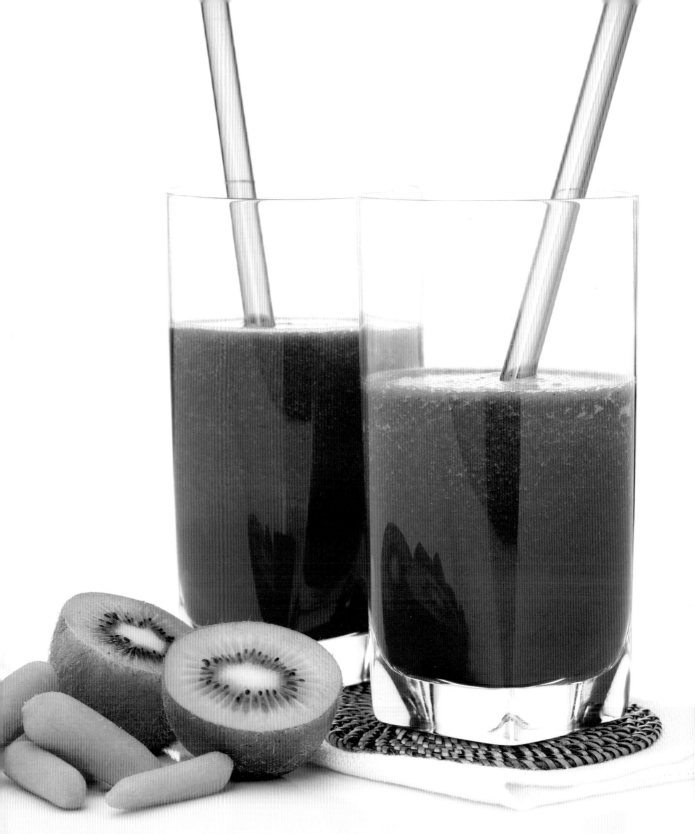

Duck Duck Gooseberry
— recipe on page 112

Chapter 3

Phytochemicals in Health and Disease

I F YOU STROLL DOWN the dietary supplement aisle of any big-box store or your local pharmacy, you'll probably notice that the labels on most of the bottles lining the shelves have long and often hard-to-pronounce names. The days of only finding actual essential nutrients, such as vitamin C and iron, are long gone. So what are most of these compounds that everyone from Madison Avenue marketers to nutrition scientists say you need to be healthy? In a word, phytochemicals — or as some prefer, phytonutrients — compounds found mainly in plants that may have some action in the human body. How many are there? Estimates run up to 10,000, and many may be yet undiscovered.

One useful distinction to keep in mind is that these compounds appear to be beneficial to health, but they are not essential, as are the essential nutrients. Phytochemicals are often referred to by scientists as bioactive, which just means they have some type of activity in the body. Although not limited to their three major roles in the body, many of the potential benefits of these compounds center around these roles, which include antioxidant, anti-inflammatory and hemodynamic effects. Most of the major chronic diseases that afflict humans, such as cardiovascular disease, diabetes and cancer, involve these actions.

While many phytochemicals can be helpful to prevent disease, not all are beneficial. One example of phytochemicals causing problems relates to a group known as goitrogens, found in cabbage and other vegetables. Goitrogens interfere with the body's thyroid hormone, and this could cause a goiter. Cooking foods inactivates goitrogens, so it's typically not a problem. However, it illustrates a key point about the phytochemicals that scientists who study toxins — toxicologists — tell us: Plant foods contain thousands of compounds, and some may be beneficial, but some are potentially toxic.

There are 10 categories of phytochemicals that may be important in chronic disease, although some of these are subsumed under another category (see Figure 1). The three major categories are flavonoids, stilbenes/lignans and phenolic acids. Of these, the flavonoids are the most diverse and have accumulated the greatest amount of evidence pointing to the strongest link to disease prevention. The flavonoids contain phytochemicals that continue to make headlines, including quercetin, a flavonol found in apples and onions, which studies have shown to be a potent anti-inflammatory agent.

In considering the importance of these phytochemicals, which are not essential nutrients, a logical question is, how do scientists determine whether a compound is a true nutrient? And how do they figure out how much we need? We'll answer the second question in the next section, on Dietary Reference Intakes (DRIs), the current nutrient standards (see opposite). As for the first question, scientists conduct various types of studies that include the use of animals. To test a specific compound to find out whether it is essential, they feed the lab animals a diet that doesn't include it. If the animal grows normally, the compound is not necessary for life, or not essential. However, if the animal displays an adverse effect consuming a diet devoid of the compound, and the effect is determined to be a symptom of deficiency, then the compound might be essential. This type of study, and of course in humans, too, is also how they determine the amounts of essential nutrients that we need.

The Yardstick: Dietary Reference Intakes (DRIs)

The nutrient intake standards, DRIs, provide an estimate of the amount of specific essential nutrients, as well as some nonessential nutrients, a healthy person needs on a daily basis. It's important to know how these intake levels are determined. The DRIs are developed by the US Institute of Medicine (IOM) under the National Academy of Sciences (NAS) and are used by the United States and Canada. One important fact to know about the NAS is that while it's a government agency, the committee that develops the DRIs consists of independent

Figure 1: Phytochemical Categories

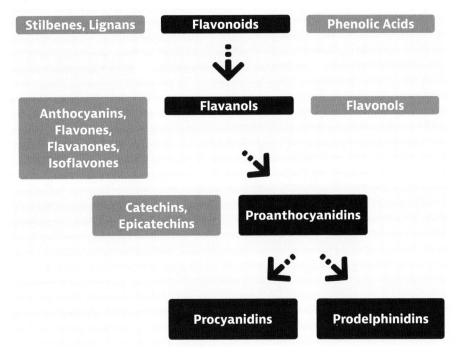

researchers representing various specialties in nutrition. This is crucial to ensure that the DRIs reflect the most current, diverse and unbiased science available.

Here's how it works: The committee reviews the latest research from various types of reports, including animal, human population and human subject studies. From this they develop an estimate of how much of a particular nutrient would meet the needs of half the population in a certain age and gender group. Recognizing that the level they recommend needs to be applicable to almost every healthy person, up to 98% of the population, they add a bit extra to the number, often referred to as a "margin of safety." This margin of safety takes into account the individual variation from person to person, as well as the variation in absorption rates of a nutrient from different foods. On the downside, the margin of safety means that the number may be higher than the level you need, so it's important to keep in mind that it's just an estimate.

Food Labeling Standards

Older versions of the DRIs are still the basis for food labeling, although the food labels will be updated in the near future to reflect the updated DRIs. In the recipe sections, the nutrition analysis shown is based on the current labeling standards, the Daily Values (DVs). Here's where it gets a bit dicey: The DVs consist of the Reference Daily Intakes (RDIs) and the Daily Reference Values (DRVs). In turn, the RDIs are an old version of labeling standards based on the recommended intakes for essential nutrients from the 1960s. While it may seem like using something that dated doesn't make sense, consider that manufacturers don't know who is eating the product, a child, an adult or a senior, so precision in labeling is not really necessary.

The DRVs are labeling standards for eight nutrients: total fat, saturated fat, cholesterol, total carbohydrates, dietary fiber, protein, potassium and sodium. Putting the DRVs and the RDIs together, we get the DVs. In the recipe section, you'll get the information that's most useful to you — how much of your daily need for a particular nutrient does the entry provide, expressed as a percentage. So, for example, many of the recipes provide 200% of the DV for vitamin A and 150% of the DV for vitamin C. This means that drinking this tasty treat gives you double the vitamin A you need for the entire day, and one and a half times more of the vitamin C you need.

Another Way to Evaluate Foods: Nutrient Density

These days, when experts tell us that overweight and obese people now outnumber those at a healthy weight, we need to look at food differently than we did in the past. A concept that dates back to the 1980s is an idea whose time has arrived — nutrient density. Simply stated, nutrient density considers the nutrients a food provides per calorie. While experts are still hashing out the ideal way to characterize foods using various scoring systems, consumers can think in terms of getting the most nutrients and phytochemicals for the least calories.

As a dietitian, when I teach this concept, I use the example of the purchasing power of your money. If you're going to purchase a new tablet, you'll most likely compare all the different tablets that are available, the features they offer, and then the price of each product. You obviously want to get the best tablet with the most features for the least amount of money. Using this same logic, comparing a 100-calorie portion of two foods, the item that gives you twice the fiber is a better deal. I generally tell clients to look for double digits for DVs, because that's the indication that a food you're evaluating is a good or excellent source of a particular nutrient.

For example, let's say you're comparing two bread products. Product A provides 4 grams of fiber per serving of 100 calories and product B contains 1 gram of fiber for that same serving. Product A's fiber content represents 16% of the DV for fiber, while product B's fiber value is only 4% of the DV. You'll notice that almost all the entries in the recipe section are nutrient dense. Since there are no standards for the beneficial phytochemicals, each entry will have a notation about the specific phytochemical it contains.

Chronic Diseases Linked to Diet and Nutrition

Overview

The major diseases that afflict modern humans, and certainly those in the top leading causes of death, include cardiovascular disease (CVD), diabetes and cancer. In North America, CVD and cancer together account for about 75% of all deaths every year. Diabetes is not only a leading cause of death, it contributes to both CVD and cancer. For all these conditions, nutrition and diet are implicated in both the cause and, at least in the case of the first two, the cornerstone of treatment. Recent research has shown that some of the processes involved in these diseases are similar. For example, scientists have known for some time that oxidative damage plays a key role in CVD and cancer, and more recently have suggested that it may also be important in diabetes. Oxidative damage and inflammation are two important processes associated with the top chronic diseases, so let's take a short detour that's important to understand how food can help protect us against these diseases. Some of this information may be familiar from high school chemistry class.

Oxidative Damage: Isn't Oxygen Supposed to Be Good?

Initially, any concern with the oxidation reaction seemed limited to food technologists, who tried to find ways to prevent foods from becoming rancid and extend shelf life. More recently, scientists have pointed to oxidation as the underlying or contributing cause of disease.

While oxygen is arguably the most vital compound to life, when it comes into the body, certain problems occur. Most of the oxygen entering the cell leaves as carbon dioxide, which we exhale every time we breathe. However, a small amount is converted to water in the mitochondria, the power plant of every cell.

During this transformation, four electrons are added. And the problem comes in when an even smaller amount undergoes this process slowly, one electron at a time. Each time this happens, it gives rise to a highly unstable compound known as a reactive oxygen species (ROS), often called a free radical, although that is only one type of ROS. This ROS zips around the body wreaking havoc by damaging important structures, such as the membrane that protects every cell, and key compounds such as cholesterol and DNA. To make matters worse, there are several of these nasty radicals, some of which live in the water compartment of the body and some of which inhabit the lipid, or fat, compartment. We'll see why this is significant shortly, when we consider how antioxidants in foods help prevent this damage.

Another scary thing about these radicals is that they recruit other normal compounds in the body over to their dark side, turning the normal compounds into an ROS in a process that has been likened to a domino effect. They keep on damaging body structures and compounds and making new recruits along the way until a protector comes along to stop them — the antioxidants. Of even more interest is the idea that there is a critical balance in the body between these damaging ROS and our antioxidant defenses.

So where do the radicals and the protective antioxidants come from? Let's start with the radicals first. We are exposed to radicals through the environment, with sources such as pollution, ultraviolet radiation from the sun, infections, cigarette smoke and certain compounds found in foods. In addition, our body produces reactive substances when there has been damage from trauma, excessive exercise or our immune system, and even in the normal course of metabolism. For a bit of perspective on our exposure to radicals, one famous expert, Bruce Ames, estimated that each one of us takes over 10,000 oxidative hits every day. So how do we manage to survive this continual attack?

Fortunately, we have several systems inside the body to protect cells and their vital structures from ROS damage, including special antioxidant enzymes and proteins. In addition, we have high-powered weapons in our arsenal — the antioxidant nutrients and phytochemicals we eat, hopefully every day. Together with the body's antioxidant network, this is termed our antioxidant defense system. If we're healthy and our diet contains an abundance of nutrient-dense foods, our antioxidant defense system will be more than adequate to protect us against those 10,000 hits!

Antioxidants in Food

The antioxidant nutrients that are essential include vitamin C and vitamin E. In addition, some phytochemicals called carotenoids, mostly beta-carotene, which gives carrots their orange color and can be converted to vitamin A, are powerful antioxidants. These nutrients stop the ROS by becoming oxidized themselves, in effect sacrificing themselves and breaking the chain of oxidation. Importantly, vitamin C, which is water soluble, acts in the water-soluble compartments of the body to protect against ROS. Vitamin E and the carotenoids are fat soluble, so they protect in the fat-soluble parts of the body.

Besides the carotenoids, many other phytochemicals are potent antioxidants. For example, flavonoids found in foods such as fruits, vegetables, coffee, chocolate and tea, and lignans found in flaxseed and sesame seeds, rival (and in some cases exceed) the antioxidant power of vitamins C and E. Since some are fat soluble and some are water soluble and vary in their potency, they complement not only the body's antioxidant system but one another as well. Numerous population studies, called epidemiologic studies, have reported that consumption of fruits and vegetables is associated with a lowered risk for various diseases. The protective antioxidants in foods have been linked to protection against CVD, diabetes, cancer and the aging process itself. And juicing makes it easier for people to regularly consume a wide variety of fruits and vegetables containing not just the antioxidant nutrients but also a diversity of healthy phytochemicals.

Inflammation

A more recent finding is that the process of inflammation, or the inflammatory response, inside the body's tissues plays a pivotal role in the development of many chronic diseases. A simple definition for what is a complex response of the body to many types of harm is that inflammation is a nonspecific, or shotgun, response to injury or infection representing a type of immune response. It's the body's attempt to protect itself from various dangers, but as with many of the body's protective measures, it can actually harm the body if the response is excessive or sustained.

To learn how inflammation is linked to chronic disease, let's look at what goes on in the process. Bacteria that sneak into the human body are a common trigger for the inflammatory response. The immune system includes specialized cells that are different types of white blood cells, tissues, compounds and organs that mount a coordinated defense to bacteria that have entered, say, through a cut in the finger. The body's first step is to detect the foreign invader and try to destroy it immediately. In addition, the immune system is alerted to the threat by these watchdog cells.

Part of the response includes dilating blood vessels leading to the injury or invasion site, in this case the finger. This allows for more blood to flow to the site and the blood vessels leading away from the site are constricted, preventing blood flow away from the area. These and other changes help limit the spread of the infection to other parts of the body while at the same time rushing immune cells to the battle to help fight the invaders. The first cells to do battle are phagocytes,

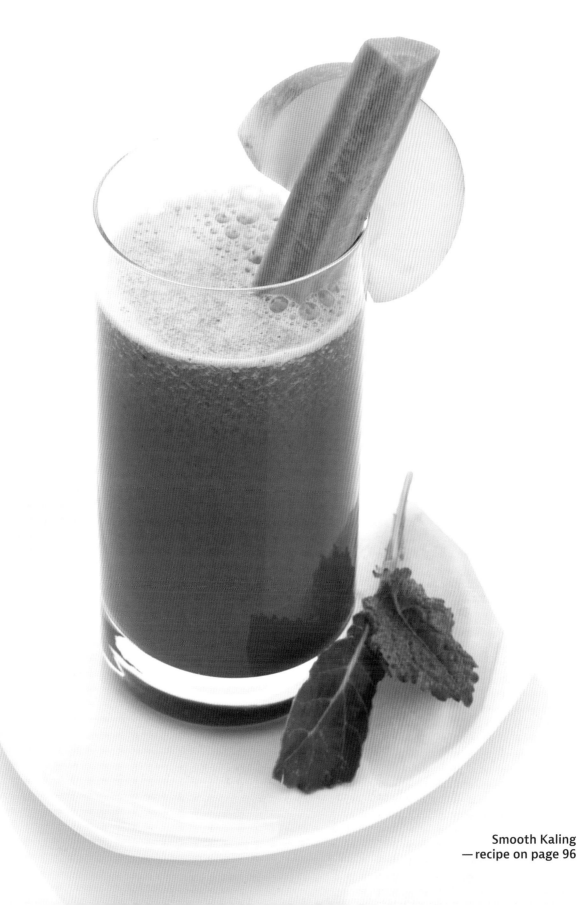

Smooth Kaling
— recipe on page 96

which gobble up the bacteria and kill them with compounds that include ROS. And the changes cause what you see and feel happening — swelling, redness, heat and pain. This counterattack by the body, the inflammatory process, helps fight the invaders, but if it becomes chronic, these cells and the compounds they release damage healthy tissue.

Inflammation and Diet

In much the same way that foods, specifically the nutrients and phytochemicals they contain, can either promote oxidative damage or protect against it, the same appears to be true for inflammation. Some of the anti-inflammatory compounds may exert their effect in a particular step of the process, but the evidence is sound that they can have an overall effect, whether beneficial or harmful, on inflammation. We'll see that the typical foods used in juicing fall on the healthy side of the inflammation equation.

As you might expect, foods that appear to promote inflammation are those that most of us should be reducing in our diet for other health reasons (see Table 5). Some of these include foods that are high in sugar and low-fiber starchy foods. These foods are often referred to as high glycemic index (or response) foods because they raise the level of sugar in the blood quickly. Other foods that promote inflammation include meats that have been char-grilled. This cooking process causes the formation of harmful compounds called advanced glycosylation end products (AGEs). These compounds are also specifically linked to cancer, based on numerous studies.

And the last category, or at least the last of those thus far determined, are foods that contain trans-fatty acids, more popularly known as trans fats. This type of fat mostly arises from the commercial process of hydrogenation. In this process, liquid oil, such as soy oil, undergoes the chemical addition of hydrogen atoms. The positioning of these hydrogen atoms is different from their position in the oil and it results in a hardened or solid fat, such as margarine. Most government agencies have mandated that products containing trans fats be labeled, since research shows that these fats are linked to many chronic diseases.

Table 5: Foods and Inflammation

Foods and Compounds that Promote Inflammation
High-sugar foods
Low-fiber starch foods
Charred meats, fish, poultry (advanced glycoslylation end products)
Hydrogenated oil (trans fats)

Foods and Compounds that Fight Inflammation
Fatty fish — salmon, mackerel, tuna (omega-3 fats)
Nuts — especially walnuts, flax seeds, chia seeds (alpha linolenic acid)
Coffee, tea
Spices — curry, ginger
Alcoholic beverages
Fruits — especially grapes and berries
Vegetables — especially celery and garlic
Whole grains
Olive oil (oleocanthal)
Unsweetened cocoa and dark chocolate (polyphenols)
Foods containing magnesium
Foods high in vitamin C
Foods high in vitamin E
Foods high in carotenoids

On the plus side of the ledger, you'll find many of the foods we have used in the recipes. Not surprisingly, most fruits and vegetables, with some exceptional standouts, are first on the list. In reviewing the research, we find some studies show specific compounds confer the anti-inflammatory effect but, in other cases, it is the food itself. One example is the entire group of berries, with studies showing a potent anti-inflammatory effect, and blueberries seem exceptional; researchers have identified several important phytochemicals, including anthocyanins, flavonols, flavanols, allotannins, proanthocyanidins, and phenolic acids.

Other inflammation-fighting foods include specific dietary fatty acids: the omega-3 fatty acids and alpha-linolenic acid (ALA). Most people are familiar with the omega-3 fats, as their protective effects against CVD have been known for several decades. Also, many of us have tried to eat more of the foods high in these healthy fats, which are fatty types of fish like salmon, tuna and mackerel. Another type of fatty acid that fights inflammation, however, is the lesser known ALA. Good sources of ALA include flax seeds, chia seeds, lingonberries, kiwi and walnuts. You'll find some of these items in Chapter 5, "High-Impact Additives: Super Enhancers," and included in several recipes.

Specific spices, such as curry, ginger and turmeric, are also potent in fighting inflammation. Olive oil, a staple in the Mediterranean region, has strong research evidence not only for powerful anti-inflammation effects but also in preventing CVD and diabetes. In the US, the Food and Drug Administration (FDA) has permitted a health claim for olive oil, based on the strong evidence. In addition, foods high in carotenoids, vitamins C and E and magnesium help fight inflammation. As with foods containing antioxidants, juicing is notable for using foods that contain high levels of these nutrients.

And saving the best for last, more recent stars in the superfoods world, and health research A-list, include coffee, cocoa and dark chocolate, and tea. While most people aren't surprised about tea, they may be shocked by coffee and cocoa. Still, the evidence is clear that both are incredibly powerful, and this is true in fighting inflammation as well as in combating ROS — double duty! Another surprise for those who think only red wine is healthful is that any type of alcohol, when consumed in moderation, also has beneficial effects, especially with regard to CVD. One of its numerous physiologic effects is reducing inflammation.

Cardiovascular Disease

Of the chronic diseases, CVD currently claims as many lives each year as the next eight leading causes of death combined, with approximately one of every two North Americans succumbing to some form of this disease. The most common form of CVD is coronary heart disease (CHD), of which myocardial infarction (MI), or heart attack, is the single largest killer of men and women around the world. A closer look at what goes on behind the scenes in leading up to the killer final act helps to explain how foods can help protect against CVD.

The underlying process of CVD is atherosclerosis, in which fatty plaques develop in a layer of the wall of the artery. As plaques accumulate, the artery becomes constricted. If a blood clot forms and can't pass through the narrowed opening, blood flow to the heart stops, causing myocardial infarction, or heart attack. If the clot is in a vessel close to the brain, a cerebrovascular accident (CVA), or stroke, ensues. These are the two main types of CVD that account for the majority of deaths.

The process of atherosclerosis starts with the body responding to an injury to the artery, and the causes of injury include smoking, environmental pollutants, high blood pressure and the aging process. Much of the injury may be due to ROS damage from at least some of those sources. And a key factor is that LDL (low-density lipoprotein) cholesterol, sometimes called the "bad cholesterol," becomes oxidized. When this happens, LDL cholesterol causes damage to the artery and also has other harmful effects that add to the possibility of a heart attack or stroke.

Another part of the process involves inflammation, which you may recall as being the most basic way that the body responds to an injury or infection. In an attempt to heal the injured artery, the body goes through repeated cycles of injury and repair, all involving inflammation and likely leading to a clot being formed. Foods may either help prevent these steps or actually promote them, since antioxidants and anti-inflammation compounds can intervene, while some foods promote inflammation.

The strongest evidence for diet and CVD is with omega-3 fats, found in fatty fish. Not only do they counter inflammation, but they also have powerful effects on the blood and arteries. Some of these effects include making clotting cells less sticky, which means they're less likely to form clots and block blood flow in the artery. In addition, these fats promote dilation of arteries, and this also helps blood flow. Studies also show that ALA, contained in plant foods such as flax, chia and walnuts, has other beneficial effects for the heart in addition to preventing inflammation. One effect is that a certain amount of ALA is converted to the more potent omega-3 fatty acids, similar to those found in fish. Researchers also believe that ALA may have other protective actions independent of these effects.

Another way in which diet and nutrition offer protection against CVD is by lowering blood pressure, which is one of the major risk factors for both heart attack and stroke. A groundbreaking study in the 1990s, Dietary Approaches to Stop Hypertension (DASH), gave rise to a powerful regimen that helps lower blood pressure in those with hypertension. The diet was notable in that it added protective foods rather than restricting foods, which had been the typical approach. Researchers found that a diet high in fruits, vegetables and low-fat dairy products was effective in reducing blood pressure in subjects with hypertension. It is still widely promoted as one of the best therapies to both lower blood pressure and help prevent heart attack and stroke. If you think it would be hard to eat 10 servings of fruits and vegetables and 3 servings of dairy every day, juicing can make it easy. One juice serving, made with recipes in this book, provides anywhere from 3 to 5 servings of fruits and vegetables.

Cancer

Over the past decades, with escalating global environmental problems and more complex lifestyles in concert with an increased life expectancy, cancer has become the second leading cause of death in adults and children in North America, second only to CVD. Internationally, close to eight million people die of cancer every year.

The development of cancer is a complex process that is influenced by genetics and many environmental factors, including diet, with some experts suggesting that heredity accounts for only 10% of cancers, depending on the type. One large study reported in the *New England Journal of Medicine* found that among identical twins, heredity accounted for only 15% of the cancers. Experts have estimated that diet is related to up to 35% of cancers, again most likely depending on the type. For example, diet is the culprit in 70% of cancers of the colon and rectum (see Figure 2).

"Cancer" is the term for numerous highly diverse diseases, but all are characterized by unrestrained growth of cells that start out as normal. The underlying problem is that the cell loses control over normal growth. Scientists have theorized that a normal cell transforms into a cancerous cell through three stages: initiation, promotion and progression.

In initiation, something outside of the body triggers a mutation, or change, in the genes that control cell production and differentiation. These triggers may include ultraviolet radiation from the sun, radiation from X-rays and other diagnostic tests, chemicals and viruses. In addition, cancer cell development is associated with the normal aging process of cells, which is why more people die of cancer now that life expectancy is higher than in the past.

Figure 2: Contribution of Diet to Cancer and Specific Types of Cancer

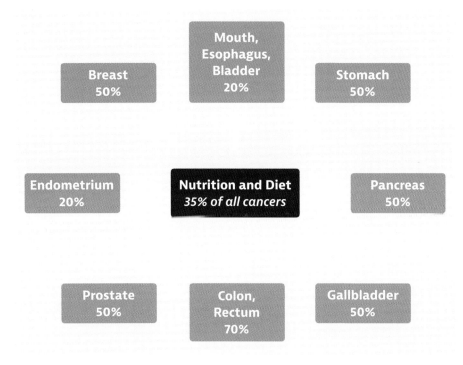

Although a mutation occurs in a cell in the initiation phase, the mutated cell may remain dormant for years. In the second phase, promotion, the dormant cell is activated — and becomes an active cancer cell — by some agent that promotes this step. Scientists believe that several agents may serve as promoters, even dietary constituents such as fat. The final phase, progression, is a series of steps that turn the cancer cell into a more malignant cell that can now spread. These steps change the genome, which is the complete set of genes in the chromosomes of each cell. The result is a cell that now divides in an uncontrolled manner, invading neighboring cells and eventually spreading far from the primary cancer.

Although scientists don't know the exact nature of carcinogenesis, or the development of cancer, they distinguish between substances that can directly cause cancer, carcinogens, and those that promote cancer. To make it more complex, not everyone exposed to the same carcinogens and promoters will have the same risk for a specific cancer. This is where genetics and nutritional factors come in yet again, in that some people will have additional protection against cancer even with exposure to carcinogens and promoters.

Oxidative Damage and Inflammation in Cancer
Researchers have provided good evidence for the theory that oxidative damage plays a key role in carcinogenesis. Laboratory studies have shown how oxidative damage to DNA leads to cancer, and it may be involved in the first two steps of the process. A person's antioxidant defense status, partly a contribution of dietary antioxidants, can influence whether they develop cancer. And indeed, numerous studies have shown that dietary and nutritional factors influence the incidence of cancer, both positively and negatively.

Some dietary factors act as carcinogens, others act as promoters, while some dietary compounds may act as anticarcinogens. One way they do this is to act as antioxidants to defend against oxidative damage. Diets high in fiber, fruits and vegetables are associated with reduced cancer risk. Researchers had first theorized that the protective compounds in fruits and vegetables were most likely vitamins E and C and carotenoids, because of their antioxidant functions. However,

Table 6: Foods Protective Against Cancer

Fruits	Vegetables	Spices, Condiments, Nuts, Seeds	Cereals, Grains, Legumes
Apple	Artichoke	Black mustard seed	Black bean
Apricot	Avocado	Black pepper	Black lentil
Banana	Broccoli	Camphor	Brown lentil
Blackberry	Brussels sprout	Cardamom	Corn
Cherry	Cabbage	Cashew nut	Green pea
Citrus fruits	Carrot	Cinnamon	Kidney bean
Dessert date	Cauliflower	Clove	Millet
Durian	Daikon	Coriander	Mung bean
Grapes	Fiddlehead	Curry leaves	Oats
Guava	Kohlrabi	Fennel	Pigeon pea
Indian gooseberry	Komatsuna (Japanese mustard green)	Fenugreek	Rice
Malay apple	Lettuce	Flaxseed	Rye
Mango	Okra	Garlic	Scarlet runner (broad) bean
Mangosteen	Onion	Ginger	Sorghum (Jowar)
Pineapple	Potato	Kalonji	Soybean
Pomegranate	Radicchio	Licorice	Wheat
	Saltbush (Orach)	Mustard seed	
	Spinach	Parsley	
	Tomato	Peanut	
	Turnip	Pecan	
	Ulluco (Andean root)	Pistachio	
	Watercress	Rosemary	
	Winter squash	Sesame seed	
	Zucchini	Star anise	
		Turmeric	
		Walnut	

Table 7: Phytochemicals Protective Against Cancer

1'-actoxychavicol acetate	Diosgenin	Mangostin
18- -glycyrrhetinic acid	Emodin	Myricetin
Acetyl-11-keto-beta-boswellic acid	Epicatechin gallate, epigallocatechin	Oleandrin
Allicin	gallate carnosol	Oleanolic acid
Alpha-lipoic acid	Epigatechin	Phenyl isothiocyanate
Alpha-tocopherol	Eugenol	Phytic acid
Anethole	Evodiamine	Piceatannol
Apigenin	Gamma-tocotrienol	Piperine
Baicalin	Garcinol	Plumbagin
Benzyl isothiocyanate	Genistein	Quinic acid
Berberine	Gingerol	Resveratrol
Beta-carotene	Glabridin	Sanguinarine
Beta-cryptoxanthine	Glycyrrhetinic acid	Sesamin
Beta-lapachone	Glycyrrhizin	Silymarin
Betulinic acid	Guggulsterone	Sulforaphane
Butein	Indiruibin-3'-monoxime	Tanshinones iia, tanshinones i
Caffeic acid phenethyl ester	Indole 3-carbinol	Theaflavin-33'-digallate
Capsaicin	Kahweol	Thymoquinone
Carnosol	Linalol	Ursolic acid
Celastrol	Lupeol	Wogonin
Chlorophyll	Lutein	Yakuchinone A, yakuchinone B
Curcumin	Lycopene	Zerumbone
Dibenzoylmethane	Mangiferin	

subsequent trials using these nutrients as supplements yielded mixed results, causing researchers to expand their search. Now it appears that numerous phytochemicals present in foods fulfill this protective role, and it's also possible that within a particular food, the compounds work together.

Although scientists have known for some time that inflammation played a role in carcinogenesis, the possibility that anti-inflammatory compounds in food could be protective is a newer area of research. Chronic inflammation, which happens as a result of certain infections (as we saw with the immune response) and also chronic diseases, significantly increases the risk for cancer. Its exact role is still the subject of study, but it appears to have several cancer-promoting effects.

One effect of inflammation, and a common link with ROS, is that when inflammation occurs as part of the immune response to an infection, the immune cells release ROS, thus delivering a carcinogenic one-two punch. Another is that inflammation is part of the process to repair tissue injuries. While it's necessary, if it keeps recurring or is chronic, inflammation promotes the formation of tumors, including those that are malignant.

The evidence is clear that specific foods are protective against cancer, whether the protection is from an anti-inflammatory, anti-oxidant or other action (see Table 6). And in some cases, studies have identified specific phytochemicals contained in foods that are involved in the anticarcinogenic effects (see Table 7).

Obesity and Inflammation

Obesity, an increasingly common condition around the world, has strong ties to several chronic diseases. Even when it doesn't play a role in actually causing a disease, it can make the disease more serious. Diseases with links to obesity, and in some cases a stronger connection, include heart disease, high blood pressure, diabetes and certain cancers.

Recent research has focused on how chronic inflammation is involved in obesity, especially when the extra weight is at or above the waistline. Obesity experts believe that the body's immune cells see the extra fat deposited in fat cells as foreign invaders. This case of mistaken identity causes the full immune response, as if there actually was a foreign invader like a virus. Special white blood cells come to the site and get caught up in the fat tissue. They release several chemicals that cause inflammation. The more fat tissue present, the higher the level of chemicals released to keep the process of inflammation going.

Diabetes

We tend to think of diabetes as a disease affecting modern humans, but it was recognized by both the early Greeks and Egyptians as far back as 1552 BCE. The Greek physician Aretaeus gave the disease its name, which translated as "to flow through a siphon," recognizing the excess urination and loss of sugar into urine. Today, diabetes exacts a tremendous toll, affecting over 25 million people in the US alone. Diabetes is the leading cause of kidney failure, amputations and new cases of blindness, and it significantly increases the risk for CVD.

Diet has always been a cornerstone of treatment, even dating back to the ancient Greeks. More recently, researchers have pointed to oxidative damage and inflammation as key features of the disease, and therefore a link to diet in its development. In the case of inflammation, researchers noted this link to diabetes, but they didn't know which came first, the inflammation or the diabetes.

The major form of diabetes, type 2, is strongly associated with obesity and insulin resistance. In insulin resistance, the pancreas produces insulin, often too much, but it is not effective in regulating blood glucose and levels rise. Obesity promotes insulin resistance in susceptible people, so this is one reason why obesity plays a role in diabetes. But the question about inflammation was whether the inflammation in obesity played a role in the development of diabetes.

A potential answer comes from a study in mice, in which researchers bred mice that could not make specific immune cells. The mice received a special diet to cause obesity, which should have also caused inflammation. However, without the special immune cells, no inflammation occurred and no insulin resistance or diabetes developed. The researchers concluded that the inflammatory response itself first causes insulin resistance, which then produces diabetes. The effect is independent of the obesity. Although this provides some good evidence, mice are not humans, so the search continues, with many researchers now testing this theory in people.

Good evidence also exists for the role of oxidative damage in diabetes, and in this case type 1 diabetes. In this form of diabetes, which usually strikes in childhood, the insulin-producing cells of the pancreas are destroyed, so no insulin is available to process carbohydrate. It appears that the same destructive ROS seen in other diseases kill pancreas cells. As with those other diseases involving ROS, improving our antioxidant defense system by eating foods high in antioxidants can lower the risk for type 1 diabetes.

If you have diabetes and want to try juicing, you will need to experiment with the effects of various types of juices on your blood glucose level. The reason why this is important has to do with this basic principle: If you compare the effect of drinking orange juice versus eating an orange on your blood glucose, the juice will cause your blood glucose to rise much more quickly than eating the orange.

Both the juice and the orange contain the same amount of naturally present sugar, but there are several reasons for the different effects on your blood glucose level. First, the juice doesn't contain as much fiber as the orange, and the fiber slows the rate of digestion and absorption of the sugars in the orange. In addition, the liquid juice gets into your digestive system more quickly than the solid orange, which requires more time for digestion, and therefore the sugar from the juice gets into your bloodstream sooner.

Of the two main types of juicing, using the blender or food processor rather than an actual juice machine will incorporate more fiber into your recipe. Also, fruits contain more sugar compared to vegetables, so the higher the proportion of fruit in a recipe, the more rapidly it will be digested and absorbed.

One other consideration is that the addition of protein-containing foods, such as yogurt, seeds, nuts or legumes, will also help slow the glycemic response. In the final analysis, though, you should track the effect of particular recipes on your blood glucose and either change the recipe (by adding yogurt, beans, nuts) or avoid those that have an adverse effect on your blood glucose level.

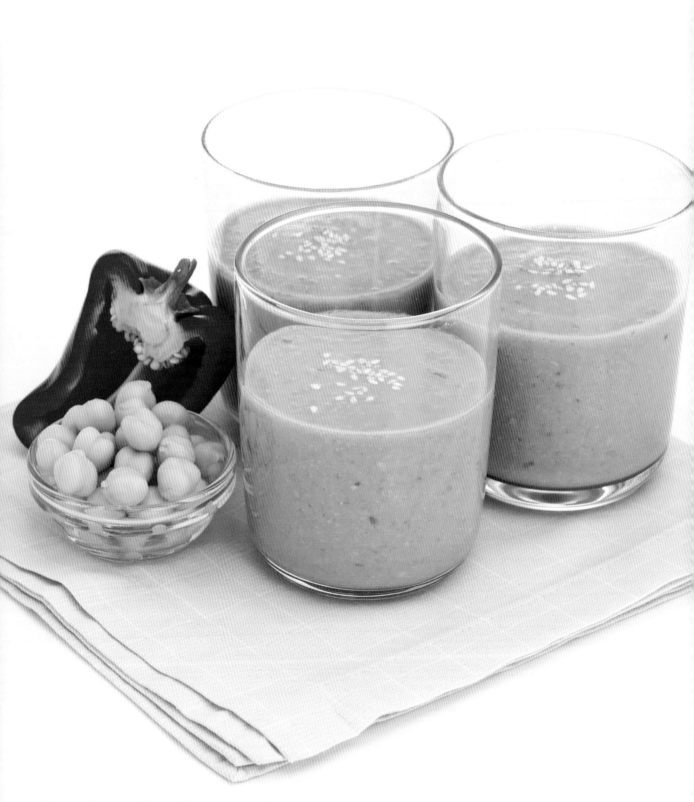

Pepper Hummus Smoothie
— recipe on page 214

Chapter 4

High-Impact Additives: Super Enhancers

Rightly or wrongly, the word "additive" doesn't exactly have the best connotations, so to emphasize the nutritional benefit of ingredients to consider adding to your juices, we've used "super enhancers." In this chapter, we'll look at some of these super enhancers and discuss their nutritional virtues and suggest some optimal uses in your recipes. In most cases, however, they will significantly change the taste of the final product, so individual preferences should still rule the day. In addition, it's important to note that even a potentially beneficial and natural substance can be harmful in high doses.

One example is cinnamon, which contains powerful antioxidant compounds but in high doses can cause liver damage. In other words, as with even essential vitamins, more is not necessarily better. An excellent resource for assessing the potential benefits and possible harmful effects of some of these substances is the US National Institutes of Health National Center for Complementary and Alternative Medicine (nccam.nih.gov).

The super enhancers fall into several categories and, in some cases, they are difficult to categorize. In general, the categories include herbs and spices, nuts and seeds, flavorings and nutrient supplements. The main benefit for most of the super enhancers, in addition to enhancing the taste of the products, is to incorporate healthy phytochemicals for added nutritional benefit. Some of the super enhancers will taste best in sweet juices and shakes, while others will work better in savory juices and sauces. Chapter 6 will give you some suggestions for using the super enhancers, but what follows provides brief descriptions and a table you can use for quick reference (see Table 8, page 70).

Herbs and Spices

Basil

Usually associated with Mediterranean cuisines, basil is a leafy herb with several cultivars used around the world in cooking and as a medicinal plant. Not only is basil high in phytochemicals, it also a good source of vitamins and minerals, such as vitamins A, C and K and manganese. Phytochemicals in basil include caffeic acid, limonene, beta sitosterol, (E)-beta-carophyllene (BCP) and ursolic acid. Studies have shown these phytochemicals have antioxidant and anti-inflammatory effects. In addition, caffeic acid has beneficial effects on the immune system and ursolic acid exerts several anticancer effects.

Cinnamon

This aromatic spice adds a distinctive flavor to milk-based shakes, calling to mind desserts such as pumpkin and apple pie. Studies have shown that cinnamon has a beneficial effect on regulating blood glucose level, even suggesting it might be helpful for people with prediabetes and diabetes, although studies are conflicting. Cinnamon is a potent antioxidant that may help lower risk for CVD and cancer. One of the phytochemicals in cinnamon is cinnamic acid. Some of the potential health effects of this compound include protection against prostate and lung cancer, inhibition of the bacteria that causes stomach ulcers (*Helicobacter pylori*), several effects on blood glucose regulation, antioxidant activity and anticlotting effects to fight heart disease. A recent study reported that adding just 1 tsp (5 mL) of cinnamon to the diet each day, which is easy to do with several of our recipes, prevented the formation of abnormal proteins in the brain that lead to Alzheimer's disease.

Garlic

This small bulb is perhaps the most loved and despised of all the superfoods. Its putative curative powers are legendary, and researchers now have the scientific tools to sift through the fact and folklore. Garlic contains essential nutrients such as vitamins C and B6 and manganese. But its content of phytochemicals has stirred the most interest, and these compounds include allyl methyl trisulfide, diallyl sulfide, allicin, limonene, oleanolic acid and methiin. The studies have shown antioxidant and anti-inflammatory effects, as well as anticlotting effects to protect against heart attack. The benefits appear to extend to cancer, with one study showing lower rates of endometrial cancer at higher intakes of the bulb.

Ginger

As with many herbs and spices, ginger has a long and storied history of use as a medicinal compound. Researchers now know that it contains several phytochemicals with potential effects on health, such as antioxidant and anti-inflammatory effects. These phytochemicals include limonene, gingerol, 6-dehydrogingerdione (DGE), shogaols and oxalic acid. Based on the antioxidant and anti-inflammatory effects, some of the studies have shown that ginger may offer protection against CVD and cancer. In addition, ginger may protect against heart disease by improving blood cholesterol levels. Pregnant women have been using ginger to counter nausea, and it may even be helpful with the nausea associated with chemotherapy.

Oregano

There is perhaps no herb more well known than oregano, no doubt because of its association with both Italian and Greek cuisine. While many people recognize the taste of oregano in pizza sauce, they may not know of its potent health benefits. Some of the interesting phytochemicals in oregano include carvacrol, ursolic acid and caffeic acid. These phytochemicals exert antioxidant and anti-inflammatory effects. In addition, carvacrol exhibits antimicrobial effects, keeping bacteria from invading our cells, and ursolic acid may protect against cancer.

Parsley

Most people think of parsley as a decorative sprig to push to the side of their plate, but this herb is a nutritional powerhouse. It can be used as a green in salads as well, not just as a seasoning herb. Parsley is loaded with nutrients, including vitamins A (as carotenoids), C and K and many essential minerals. In addition, it's bounty of phytochemicals includes aopiole, apigenin, luteolin and rutin. This combination provides anti-inflammatory, antioxidant and anticancer health benefits.

Rosemary

Another highly aromatic herb, rosemary is notable for a high number and level of phytochemicals. Some of these include carnosic acid, rosmarinic acid, camphor, caffeic acid, ursolic acid, betulinic acid, rosmaridiphenol and rosmanol. As with the other herbs, all these compounds exhibit either anti-inflammatory or antioxidant protection. Researchers have cited one phytochemical in particular, carnosic, as being especially active in protecting the brain against diseases affecting that organ, such as Alzheimer's.

Turmeric

Turmeric is one of the most widely studied spices, with convincing evidence for its health benefits. The main phytochemical that is under study is curcumin. Originally thought to be mainly a powerful antioxidant, evidence now points to numerous effects that include antimicrobial, anti-inflammatory and several anticancer effects. Several studies showed that turmeric was effective in reducing osteoarthritis pain, and one study showed it to be as effective as anti-inflammatory drugs.

Flavorings

Cocoa Powder

Usually thought of as treats, cocoa and chocolate have a new reputation as superfoods. Extracted from the bean of the cacao tree, cocoa powder is the solid byproduct of processing the beans and removing the cocoa butter. In contrast, chocolate contains the solids and the cocoa butter, so it's high in fat, whereas cocoa powder is not. Cocoa powder makes a great additive to recipes, as it contains essential nutrients and beneficial phytochemicals. The essential minerals include potassium, copper, magnesium, manganese and zinc, and it's a good source of dietary fiber. Of more interest, though, are the phytochemicals, which include proanthocyanidins, theaflavins, catechins, cyanidins, methylxanthines and gallic acid. In fact, a study comparing beneficial phytochemicals in cocoa, tea and red wine found that cocoa had the highest content and antioxidant activity per serving — up to five times higher than black tea, up to three times higher than green tea and up to twice as high as red wine.

Soy Sauce

Most people think of soy sauce only as something to avoid because of its high sodium content. However, this soy product has been upgraded, if not to superfood status, at least to honorable mention as far as flavorings go. The traditional method of making soy sauce involves fermenting soybeans and wheat flour. Although this process reduces the level of isoflavones (phytochemicals in soybeans), it also produces other antioxidants, melanoidins, and an especially potent antioxidant, maltol. Studies have shown that maltol prevents oxidation in lab tests and in animals. A study done at the National University of Singapore showed that soy sauce contains 10 times the antioxidant level of red wine. Add soy sauce to savory juices to boost antioxidants and also enhance the other flavors. Soy sauce contains glutamate, which stimulates the umami, a savory flavor and one of the five basic tastes.

Nuts, Beans (Legumes), Seeds

Beans and Legumes

Dried beans and peas, also known as legumes and pulses, are excellent sources of many essential nutrients and important phytochemicals. Most legumes share a similar nutrient profile, so the only member of the group we'll consider separately is the soybean (see the soy entry in this category). In addition to their nutritional benefits, legumes are an excellent ingredient in juices and smoothies, as they can add depth and consistency for a truly filling beverage. You can either soak and cook the dried beans, which saves money, or, if time is limited, use canned beans for the same health benefits.

Legumes are generally good sources of protein, fiber, several B vitamins and essential minerals. They are one of the best sources of soluble fiber, which may account for study results showing that consuming beans lowers blood glucose and blood cholesterol. The phytochemicals in legumes include quercetin, saponins and inositol hexaphosphate (IP6). Studies have shown that quercetin has antioxidant and anti-inflammatory effects, as well as protecting against cancer. In addition to antioxidant activity, saponins have other anticancer effects. Researchers have studied IP6 and reported that it reduces tumor development and growth in animals, although more human study is needed.

Chia Seeds

Best known for growing green hair on pottery of Chia Pet fame, the tiny chia seed packs a powerful punch of nutrition and is a true superfood. The plant is a member of the mint family and indigenous to Central America. Chia is a good source of protein, fiber and calcium and contains omega-3 fatty acids as alpha-linolenic acid (ALA). The antioxidants in chia seeds include quercetin, caffeic acid and chlorogenic acid, which may also have other health benefits. The high fiber content in the seeds causes them to absorb water, so they can be used to thicken and add texture.

Flaxseed

Flaxseed has been used as a medicinal food for centuries. It contains many essential nutrients and phytochemicals that can be beneficial. Flaxseed is an excellent source of dietary fiber and a good source of protein, several vitamins and the minerals magnesium, potassium, iron and copper. It is also high in ALA and the phytochemicals known as lignans. Lignans are phytoestrogens, and flax contains two lignans, matairesinol and secoisolariciresinol, which are antioxidants with other anticancer effects. When using flaxseed, you should either purchase it milled, or ground, or use a food processor or a spice or coffee grinder to grind it yourself. If you use whole flaxseed, the body can't absorb the nutrients and phytochemicals.

Seed and Sprout Mixes

Several products combine the nutritional power of a variety of seeds in an easy-to-use mixture, and these convenient products can enhance your juices and smoothies. One such product, Garden of Life's Super Seed, is a proprietary blend of the sprouts from amaranth, millet, quinoa, buckwheat, chickpeas (garbanzo beans), lentils, adzuki beans, flaxseed, sunflower seeds., pumpkin seeds, chia seeds and sesame seeds. It's high in protein, fiber, omega-3 fatty acids (ALA) and, of course, plenty of phytochemicals.

Soybeans and Soybean Products

Soybeans and products made from them are a staple in certain parts of the world. They contain essential nutrients and numerous phytochemicals. Soybeans are an excellent source of dietary fiber, good-quality protein, B vitamins and several essential minerals. The phytochemicals include daidzein, genistein, glycitein, coumestrol, gallic acid, saponins, beta-sitosterol and inositol hexaphosphate. Several of these are phytoestrogens with blood-cholesterol-lowering and anti-cancer activity. Most of the phytoestrogens in soy are in the isoflavone family, and researchers have suggested possible roles in preventing CVD, diabetes, cancer and osteoporosis. Tofu is a soy product made by adding a coagulating agent (such as calcium, which also adds a vital nutrient) to soy milk and then pressing out the liquid to form a block — an ideal product to use as a superfood ingredient in juices and shakes.

Walnuts and Other Nuts

Almost all nuts are loaded with essential nutrients and numerous healthful phytochemicals, so they boost nutrition when they're added to recipes. The only caveat is that they also add significant calories, so you will want to use them judiciously if you are trying to lose weight.

Since all nuts share a similar nutrient profile, we'll focus on walnuts, as the research shows them to be one of the best nuts for health. Like most tree nuts, the main types of fat in walnuts are polyunsaturated and monounsaturated. These fats are associated with protection against heart disease. In addition, walnuts are high in alpha-linolenic

Table 8: Super Enhancers

	Nutrients and Phytochemicals	Potential Health Benefits
Herbs and Spices		
Basil	Vitamins A, C, K, manganese, caffeic acid, limonene, beta sitosterol, (E)-beta-carophyllene, ursolic acid	Antioxidant, anticancer, strengthen immune system
Cinnamon	Cinnamic acid, tannins, flavonoids, glycosides, terpenoids, coumarin, anthraquinones	Insulin effects, antioxidant, stomach protection, anticancer, anticlotting
Garlic	Vitamins C, B6, manganese, allyl methyl trisulfide, diallyl sulfide, allicin, limonene, oleanolic acid, methiin	Antioxidant, anti-inflammatory, anticlotting, anticancer effects
Ginger	Limonene, gingerol, 6-dehydrogingerdione (DGE), shogaols, oxalic acid	Anti-nausea, antioxidant, anti-inflammatory, anticlotting, anticancer effects
Oregano	Carvacrol, ursolic acid, caffeic acid	Antimicrobial, antioxidant, anti-inflammatory, anticlotting, anticancer effects
Parsley	Vitamins A (as carotenoids), C, K, essential minerals, aopiole, apigenin, luteolin, rutin	Anti-inflammatory, antioxidant, anticancer effects
Rosemary	Carnosic acid, rosmarinic acid, camphor, caffeic acid, ursolic acid, betulinic acid, rosmaridiphenol, rosmanol	Anti-inflammatory, antioxidant
Turmeric	Curcumin	Antioxidant, antimicrobial, anti-inflammatory, several anticancer effects; reduce osteoarthritis pain
Flavorings		
Cocoa powder	Potassium, copper, magnesium, manganese, zinc, fiber, proanthocyanidins, theaflavins, catechins, cyanidins, gallic acid, methylxanthines	Antioxidant, anti-inflammatory, anticlotting effects
Soy sauce	Melanoidins, maltol	Antioxidant

Table 8 (continued): Super Enhancers

	Nutrients and Phytochemicals	Potential Health Benefits
Nuts, Beans (Legumes), Seeds		
Beans	Protein, fiber, soluble fiber, several B vitamins, essential minerals, quercetin, saponins, inositol hexaphosphate	Antioxidant, anti-inflammatory, anticancer effects
Chia seeds	Protein, fiber, calcium, omega-3 fatty acids (ALA), quercetin, caffeic acid, chlorogenic acid, ferulic acid	Antioxidant, anti-inflammatory, anticancer effects
Flaxseed	Protein, fiber, magnesium, potassium, iron, copper, ALA, lignans (matairesinol, secoisolariciresinol)	Antioxidant, anti-inflammatory, anticancer effects
Seed and sprout mix	Protein, fiber, ALA, various phytochemicals from all seeds used	Antimicrobial, antioxidant, anti-inflammatory, anticlotting, anticancer effects
Soybeans	Protein, B vitamins, fiber, essential minerals, daidzein, genistein, glycitein, coumestrol, gallic acid, saponins, beta-sitosterol, inositol hexaphosphate	Blood-cholesterol-lowering, anticancer activity, protect against CVD, diabetes, cancer, osteoporosis
Walnuts and other nuts	Protein, fiber, omega-3 fatty acids (ALA), manganese, copper, magnesium, vitamin B6, thiamin, folate, beta-sitosterol, ellagic acid, myricetin	Blood-cholesterol-lowering, anticancer (prostate, pancreatic) effects
Nutrition Supplements		
Spirulina and algae	Protein, vitamins C, E, K, B vitamins, copper, iron, manganese, magnesium, potassium, beta-carotene, other antioxidants	Blood pressure and blood-cholesterol-lowering, CVD, antioxidant, anticancer. anti-inflammatory effects
Whey protein	Protein, calcium, potassium, bioactive compounds	Anti-inflammatory, antioxidant, anticancer, immune-enhancing effects, aid weight loss

acid (ALA), a plant source of omega-3 fatty acids that have a special role in preventing heart disease. Other essential nutrients in walnuts include manganese, copper, magnesium, vitamins B6, thiamin and folate. Walnuts are also a good source of dietary fiber and protein. The phytochemicals in walnuts include phytosterols, and especially beta-sitosterol, ellagic acid and myricetin. All these have antioxidant activity, and studies show that myricetin lowered risk for prostate and pancreatic cancer. In addition to antioxidant activity, ellagic acid also had other anticancer effects, and studies have shown that beta-sitosterol lowers blood cholesterol levels.

Nutrition Supplements

Spirulina and Other Algae

Often thought of as a nuisance in pool water, certain members of the algae family are actually superfoods. Many ancient cultures harvested algae from their coastlines, and it served as an excellent source of nutrients. Spirulina is a specific type of blue-green algae known as cyanobacteria. It can be a great addition to your juices and smoothies, and it's easy to add either in flake or powder form to your recipes.

Spirulina is an excellent source of protein, vitamins C, E and K, several B vitamins and key minerals such as copper, iron, manganese, magnesium and potassium. It is also high in many antioxidants, and especially beta-carotene. Studies have shown a beneficial effect on blood pressure and blood cholesterol levels, pointing to protection against CVD. In addition, researchers have reported that the antioxidants and anti-inflammatory compounds in spirulina and other blue-green algae protect against cancer.

Whey Protein

If your only exposure to whey has been in the nursery rhyme about little Miss Muffet, you are in for a nutritional treat. Whey is a byproduct of cheese production, and you can buy it in powdered or liquid form. The three forms of commercial whey include whey isolate, hydrolysate and concentrate. It adds protein, calcium and potassium and much more to juices and smoothies. Researchers have identified several bioactive compounds in whey that have anti-inflammatory, antioxidant and other anticancer effects. In addition, some studies have shown an immune-boosting effect. This protein gained fame after studies reported that it could help with weight loss. One such study showed that in a comparison between different types of proteins, whey protein affected hormones to suppress appetite and food intake.

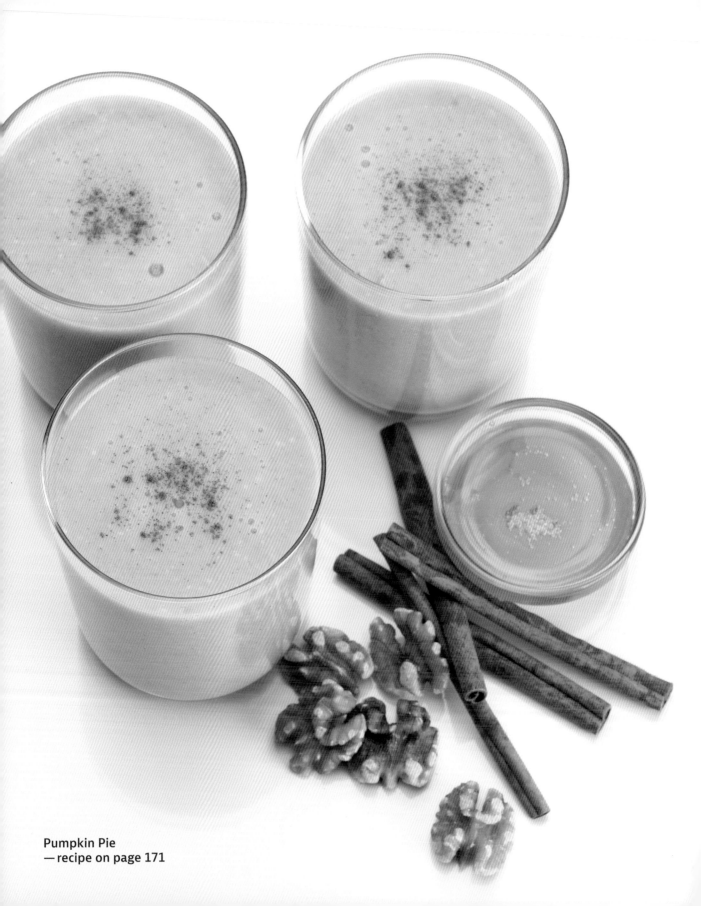

Pumpkin Pie
— recipe on page 171

Chapter 5

The How-To of Juicing

How Do I Know What Type Of Juicer I Need?

Blenders and juicers come in a wide variety of shapes and sizes. There is no single machine that will do everything well, so you may need more than one, depending on what you want to do. We'll discuss the pros and cons of several machines to help you get a better idea of what may be the best choice for you and cover the most common types of machines for home use: blenders, centrifugal juicers, masticating and auger juicers, wheatgrass juicers and citrus juicers.

Blenders

The blender is by far the oldest such machine in the kitchen, having been around since the early 20th century. In the late 1930s, Fred Waring, of Big Band fame, founded the Waring Company. Waring improved and widely marketed the blender, which was called the Miracle Mixer and later renamed the Waring Blendor.

Blenders are a quick and inexpensive way to begin juicing. The mechanism is relatively simple, it's easy to clean, it's very easy to use, and you most likely have one already. The beauty of using a blender to make smoothies (you can't really "juice" with a blender, since it's only mode of operation is to purée and blend) is that you get all the nutritional benefits of whatever goes into it. While a juicer extracts juice from fruits and vegetables, it leaves behind the often fiber-rich pulp and skin of produce. With a blender, there's much less waste and much more fiber. You can also mix in ice for a refreshing summer smoothie.

The bottom part of the blender is called the housing. This is where the brains of the operation are located. It contains the control pad, switch or buttons and the motor. The motors typically vary from about 300 watts to as many as 1500 watts. The housing may be made from plastic, stainless steel or a variety of other materials. If the blender is going to be left out on a counter, you will want to choose something that will complement your décor. The blade fits into the motor spindle and is housed inside a collar with a gasket to keep whatever's inside from leaking onto the housing. The blade assembly is attached to the jar, which is usually made of glass but may be made from other materials, such as stainless steel or polycarbonate. And, of course, on top is the lid, which sometimes has a removable center so that you can add ingredients to your smoothie while you're making it without spraying them all over the kitchen.

Centrifugal Juicers

Modern juicers were perfected and marketed in the 1930s by Dr. Norman Walker. The juicer that he pioneered, the Norwalk juicer, is still on the market today. The centrifugal juicer works by shredding the fruit or vegetable by means of a spinning plate. The juice is then forced through a strainer and out, and the pulp is ejected through a separate opening. Some machines have a setting for variable pulp, so that the amount of pulp in the drink can be varied. The centrifugal juicer has a base, which, like the blender, houses the motor and electronics, as well as the control panel. The upper section includes the housing, which protects the user from the spinning blades and holds the strainer basket and possibly a separate filter. The juicer may also have some type of container to catch the pulp as it is ejected. The lid contains an opening to insert the fruits and vegetables and a food pusher to force the material against the blade to be processed. This type of juicer does add some air to the juiced material, so the final product might be frothy and may not last quite as long in the refrigerator as that produced by a masticating-type juicer. These juicers work well with all types of fruits and hard or soft vegetables, but not very well with leafy vegetables or grasses. The nutritional "downside" of using a centrifugal juicer is that unless you utilize the pulp (and we have included some recipes for doing so; see All Things Pulp, page 147), you will lose much of the fiber and, potentially, small amounts of the nutrients.

Single- and Double-Auger Juicers

Juicers that extract the juice by means of an auger system, known as masticating juicers, are a very efficient means of juicing. The low speed of the auger makes these machines quieter than most centrifugal juicers, and the auger action produces less heat and less foam in the juice as well. The action also produces more juice from the same amount of material. The auger operates as a sort of press, pushing the product to be juiced against a screen and squeezing the juice out of it. This type of juicer will more efficiently juice such things as wheatgrass and leafy greens that the centrifugal juicer is either not able to juice or juices very inefficiently.

Single-auger juicers will make nut butters, grind spices and mince herbs, and may come with attachments that will extrude pasta and make soy milk, baby food, frozen desserts and even bread sticks. They are easy to clean; the parts can be rinsed and placed in the dishwasher. The double-auger juicer works on the same principle as the single-auger type, except that the material is pressed between two augers and through a screen. It produces the driest pulp; therefore, it extracts the most juice. Single- and double-auger machines have the same component parts. The largest part of the machine is the housing, which contains the motor and gears as well as the controls, the auger or augers, a screen that covers the augers, an end cap, a funnel and feed tube, and accessories such as a plunger to push the material through the feed tube, containers to catch the juice and pulp, and possibly other accessories, depending on the make and model of the juicer.

Other Types of Juicers

The slow juicer is a variation of the masticating juicer. The "slow" in the name refers to the action and speed of the juicing mechanism and not to the speed of the juicing, which is often faster than the centrifugal juicer. It works on low rpm's, as few as 80, is very efficient and takes up less counter space than the more common horizontal juicers. The principle and the parts of the machine are similar to other masticating juicers.

The wheatgrass juicer, as the name indicates, is made primarily for juicing wheatgrass and other types of grass such as lemon grass, but it also works well with leafy greens and soft vegetables. Although the masticating and auger juicers will also juice grasses, this type of machine is made specifically for the job. Wheatgrass juicers may be motor driven or hand cranked. The hand cranked variety can be clamped to your tabletop or countertop and gives you a little extra workout as a bonus.

A manual juicer, or reamer, is easily operated and is sufficient for anyone who only needs to juice an occasional orange or lemon. Citrus juicers are made specifically for all types of citrus. They are recommended for large amounts of juicing or for someone who juices citrus on a frequent basis. This type of juicer gives you everything that comes out of the fruit, including seeds and large pieces of pulp, which need to be strained out. The electric juicer is a better choice for large amounts of juice or frequent citrus juicing. On some machines, you can vary the amount of pulp from low pulp to heavy pulp. Most of these machines are very simple to operate and to clean, and most have dishwasher-safe parts for even easier cleanup.

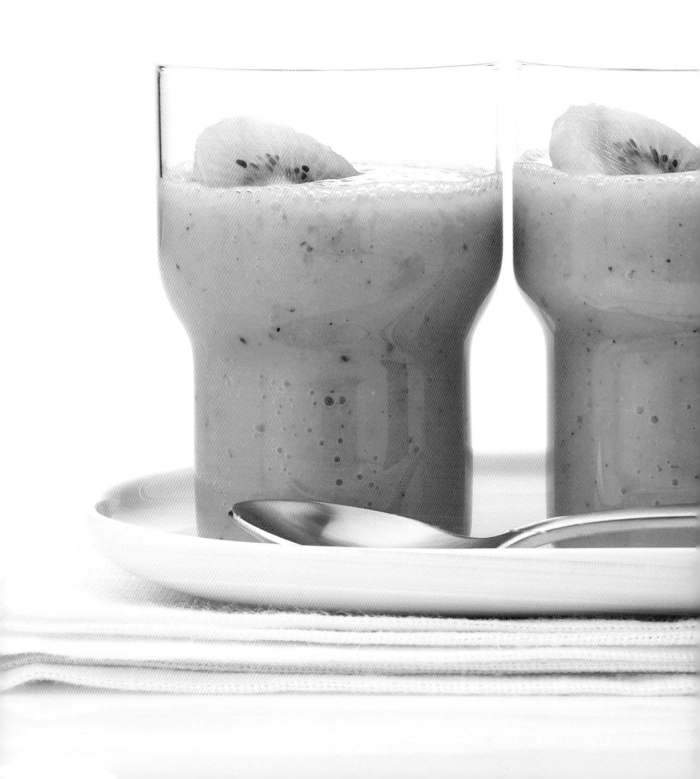

Recipes

Just Desserts Smoothie
—recipe on page 183

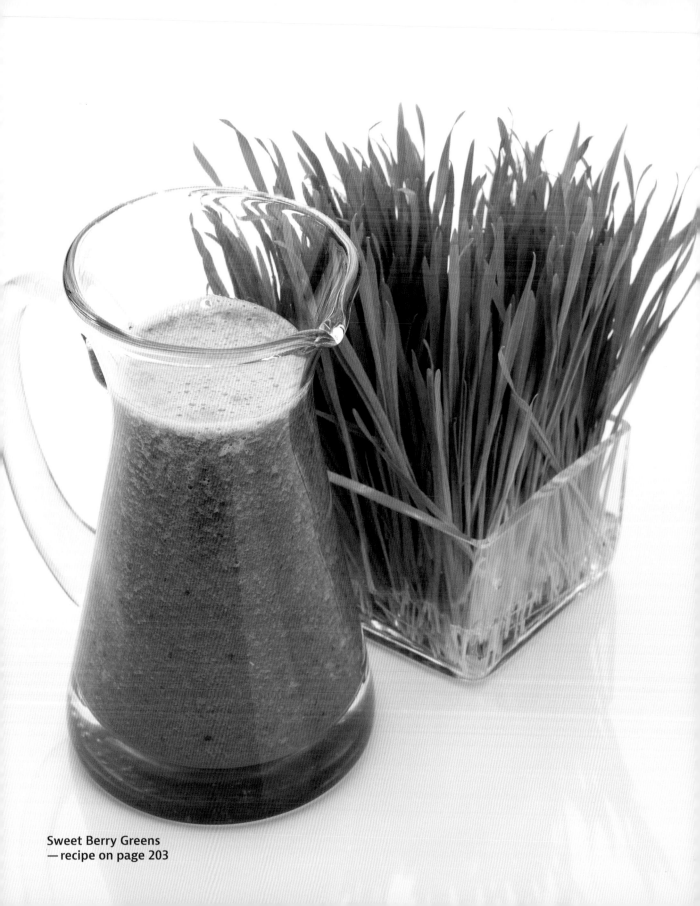

Sweet Berry Greens
— recipe on page 203

Chapter 6

Recipe Information

N EACH OF THE RECIPES, you'll notice a designation at the top of the page that indicates whether the item is prepared with a juicer or blender (or food processor). That is not to say you can't use the other machine for a particular recipe, but it will change the consistency and the nutritional analysis to some extent. In addition, we selected the ingredients for the recipes based on nutritional benefits and taste. If you are either allergic to a particular ingredient or simply have a different food preference, substituting a similar ingredient should not affect the recipe. If you don't like strawberries, for example, you can use blackberries. The dark color might not be too appetizing, but other than that, the recipe will not be adversely affected. Another personal preference is consistency. If you prefer your juices or smoothies on the thinner side, see Table 9 on page 86 for possible thinning agents.

You'll also find suggestions for super enhancers, which are superfood ingredients you can add to boost the health and nutritional benefits. One disclaimer at the outset is that many people prefer not to use certain ingredients, such as artificial sweeteners, so that may be a consideration. The research indicates that the approved sweeteners are safe, and they can be useful to replace their higher-calorie counterparts. This is helpful for people trying to lose weight or prevent weight gain.

Measurements and Nutritional Analysis

The recipes conform to how you generally see recipes presented, with both imperial and metric measures first. But since we were striving for precision in recipe amounts and in analyzing nutrition, you will notice that ingredients were also weighed. Even when using standard measures of volume, such as cups, tablespoons and mLs, some ingredients take up more or less space and volume is not the most precise measure. Take, for example, a cup (250 mL) of strawberries. Depending on the size of the individual berries, there may be more or less empty space in that cup measure. And certainly produce items vary in size; one banana, for example, can be up to double the size of another. For this reason, you'll also notice that some of the recipes give different weights for a specific fruit or vegetable for the same volume, which reflects the fact that one piece of the exact same produce varies from one purchase to another.

If you don't have a kitchen scale, it would be a worthwhile investment, not just for precision in recipes but also for assessing calories in different foods. Some scales include a built-in database that can show you the calories for the food item you are weighing. This can be a real advantage for those who either want to lose weight or make sure they don't gain weight. For units, most kitchen scales will have more than one mode, metric and imperial, or grams and ounces, respectively. We primarily used metric weights, but you can easily set your scale to whichever unit you prefer. For liquid ounces, we have shown the metric equivalent in milliliters.

Another important note relating to precision is about the nutritional analysis. For recipes using a blender or food processor, the nutritional analysis is precise and accurate, since everything put into the blender will be consumed. This is not true for recipes using a juicer. Since the juicer extracts the liquid portion of the ingredients and removes the pulp, not only is most of the fiber removed, but most of any additional nutrients contained in seeds. Seeds tend to be powerhouses of nutrients, not just for fiber but protein, vitamins and minerals.

For most produce, this is not a significant source of nutrients, but in an item containing many seeds, it is significant. Here's an example: Compare a cup of blueberries to a cup of blackberries. They seem to be quite similar, and on the surface they are, both providing about 60 to 80 calories and both chock full of important antioxidants. But a closer examination reveals that the blackberries contain more than twice the fiber and protein of the blueberries. The blackberries also contain twice the iron and four times the calcium. This is due to the presence of the large seeds in the blackberries. When the blackberries are juiced, not only is the fiber extracted but also other nutrients in the seeds, such as protein and minerals.

So here is the caveat when you consider the nutritional analysis for the juiced recipes: Since there is no truly precise way to do the analysis, short of a laboratory assessment using a gadget called a bomb calorimeter, the juiced recipe will display only the original fiber content. The reason why we included the fiber on the recipes is that if you use the pulp, which we highly encourage and provide some recipes for as well, you will obtain any nutrients the pulp contains.

Another special note about recipes relates to the yields and serving sizes. Since people vary in the amount of juice or smoothie they want to consume at one time, we used a rough standard of approximately 1 cup (250 mL) as the standard serving. However, since some recipes yield slightly more or less, when the amount is short of 2 cups (500 mL), we considered that 1 serving. The exception to this is when the calorie level is high because of the use of certain ingredients, such as mangos or bananas, or when the ingredients yield a low volume of liquid after the juicing process.

The nutrition and health information is provided in two places on each recipe page: the sidebar and the bottom. The nutrition vital stats, at the side, show the basic information: calories, protein, carbohydrate, fat and fiber. The information at the bottom shows you the percentage of the Daily Value (%DV) that 1 serving provides of essential vitamins and minerals, as well as the various phytochemicals contained in the recipe. The B vitamins are listed by their numbers: B1 (thiamin), B2 (riboflavin), B3 (niacin), B6 (pyridoxine). We didn't provide amounts of phytochemicals because that information is not available.

Blender Tips

Depending on several variables, especially the size of the blender motor, the ingredients can get jammed. A few ways around this include adding a tablespoon or two (15 to 30 mL) of water. This will generally get the blades moving again. As long as you don't add too much water,

Table 9: Thinning Agents

Thin with	Advantage
Almond or soy milk	Useful for those who are lactose intolerant or have a milk allergy; adds phytochemicals
Coconut water	Relatively low in calories, high in potassium and contains antioxidants
Coffee	A true superfood that adds numerous phytochemicals and no calories
Diet soda	Adds carbonation and many potential flavors, for example diet cream soda, and no calories
Kefir	Adds nutrients from milk and probiotics
Skim milk	Part of several enzymes, including one that fights free radicals; adds protein, calcium and numerous vitamins and minerals
Soda water	Adds carbonation and no calories
Tea	Adds phytochemicals but no calories; try green teas with different fruits, such as green tea mango, but add the tea after it has cooled
Water	No calories added

it won't significantly affect the nutritional analysis, since volume is only slightly increased. However, if you like a thicker consistency and prefer not to add water, using the stop/start button, which is usually opposite the normal blender setting, like a toggle switch can also help. And another method is to use a spatula to redistribute the ingredients, but make sure to unplug the blender for safety.

Another good tip is that if you prefer the consistency of a slushy, which is great on a hot day, you can use frozen fruits or vegetables in place of fresh. You can freeze your produce prior to processing or use a few frozen items you've purchased, especially when they are not in season. Take the case of a true superfood like sour cherries. In Michigan, where we live, they are available for about one week. If you miss that week, you don't get sour cherries. And most people don't live near orchards, so it's even more difficult to obtain these special cherries. So purchase them frozen, which is even better because they've been pitted, and plan to always keep them on hand. An alternative to using frozen produce to achieve the slushy effect is to add ice cubes.

We had a group of recipe tasters, and we soon realized that the range of individual preferences was quite wide. We did not include any recipes to which even one taster had an objection, although we did not have unanimity on how great each recipe tasted. One aspect of taste that varied the most was the desire for a sweet taste in the product. Splenda is an obvious choice for those who want sweetness without adding calories. However, some people don't want to use artificial sweeteners. You can certainly use sugar, but keep in mind it adds 15 calories per teaspoon (5 mL). Another choice is to use honey or molasses, which still add a similar level of calories but may offer some phytochemicals. You can also add a date or two, depending on how much sweetness you want. The date is a superfood that adds 20 calories but also offers phytochemicals, fiber, protein and essential minerals. We found that just one date did the sweet trick for our tasters who liked their juice on the sweet side.

Nutrition Tips

It doesn't pay to be a fresh produce purist when it comes to certain superfoods. Pumpkin, for example, is just too super to pass up, even though you will most likely not want to wait until they're available and then go through the arduous process of cleaning and cooking it. Please consider using canned pumpkin — pure pumpkin purée though, not pie filling, which is sweetened — because it's just too easy, economical, time-saving and nutrient dense to not use. Just consider that for a mere 40 calories in ½ cup (125 mL), you get 300% of the DRI for vitamin A and 20% of your daily need for fiber, not to mention lots of important phytochemicals. We've included it in a few awesome-tasting recipes that are sure to remind you of the crisp air of autumn. You'll find pumpkin in the blender recipes, since it doesn't require special processing, but you can experiment with adding a few scoops into a recipe prepared in the juicer by just whisking it into the finished juice product.

Another important nutrition tip is to leave the skins on your fruit and vegetables whenever possible. The skin on a ripe mango, for example, tastes just fine and adds key nutrients and phytochemicals. In addition, it's less work for you and there will be less waste. Of course, it's important to carefully wash produce when you don't remove the peel. Consider purchasing a good produce scrub brush, if you don't have one. And while we're on the subject of purchasing equipment, if you don't have a salad spinner, you may want one of these. Many superfoods fall within the leafy green family, such as kale, collard and other greens. They are quite difficult to clean properly, however, and the use of a spinner will ensure that dirt and insects are removed.

Leaving produce intact won't, of course, work for some items, such as citrus fruits. The rind is too bitter to include, so they need to be peeled. But as long as you remove seeds, which are extremely bitter, you can be less meticulous about removing the white fibrous material (called pith) and the membranes. These structures provide an excellent source of fiber, especially soluble fiber, and leaving them on saves you time and results in less waste of the precious juices inside the fruit. Recipes calling for lime and lemon usually recommend including only the juice. In our recipes, we include the entire slice except for the rind.

One of the best parts about juicing is the fun of trying new things. For some people, though, it's hard to envision how fruits and vegetables can work together in terms of taste. In most recipes, we've done that for you. One example is mushrooms, which are a true superfood containing essential minerals and key phytochemicals for few calories. We combined mushrooms with specific fruits that disguise the taste extremely well. If you want to try it on your own and are having a hard time figuring out how, many superfoods lend themselves to being readily disguised. These include most of the leafy greens, such as kale and romaine lettuce. They will add numerous nutrients and phytochemicals, and in the case of romaine, additional liquid. Another example is carrots, which add nutrients and phytochemicals and also impart sweetness as well as a lovely orange color.

It's easy to think of how just about any fruit will combine with another and taste wonderful. So here's a great tip for adding the nutritional power of vegetables: Make extra juice from certain vegetables, such as kale, and pour into an ice cube tray (a silicon tray is even better — you'll be able to pop one cube out at a time). When you're in a hurry, mix your fruits and then pop in a veggie cube. This is also great for boosting the nutrition of soups, sauces and chili.

And one last tip, since we mentioned being in a hurry, is to consider using produce that is easier to work with. For example, some of our recipes use carrots that you'll need to scrub and cut into pieces, and others use bagged baby carrots. The baby carrots don't seem to be as tasty as "regular" carrots, but they don't require washing, scrubbing and cutting. Another example is bagged and washed greens, such as kale, collards and romaine lettuce. They cost more, but there is no waste and no time spent in the cleaning process. So if time works against you, think about these special convenience products as a way to get the nutrition of these superfoods without the investment of time.

Food Safety Concerns

Food safety is an important consideration in any kitchen operation, but especially when combining various foods and using machines. Each of these elements introduces a potential source of risk. Food scientists often warn about cross-contamination when it comes to food safety. "Cross-contamination" refers to the introduction of microorganisms, like pathogenic bacteria, the type that can make people sick, from one food to another. The classic example is cutting raw chicken on a cutting board and then cutting a raw vegetable on the board without cleaning it. The bacteria from the chicken will now be on the vegetable. The chicken will be cooked, so that kills the bacteria on that food, but if the vegetable is eaten raw, the bacteria will end up in the unsuspecting eater's stomach.

In using juicers and blenders, if produce is not properly cleaned and the machines are not well cleaned between uses, this can be a source of bacteria. This also applies to cutting boards and other utensils, so proper cleaning of the work area is critical.

Another concern related to microbial growth is that once produce has been liquefied, bacteria have more opportunity to multiply. Juices and smoothies should be consumed soon after blending. Depending on the specific ingredients, you can probably still use a beverage the next day if it has been refrigerated at the appropriate temperature; yet the safest way to store it is to freeze unused portions.

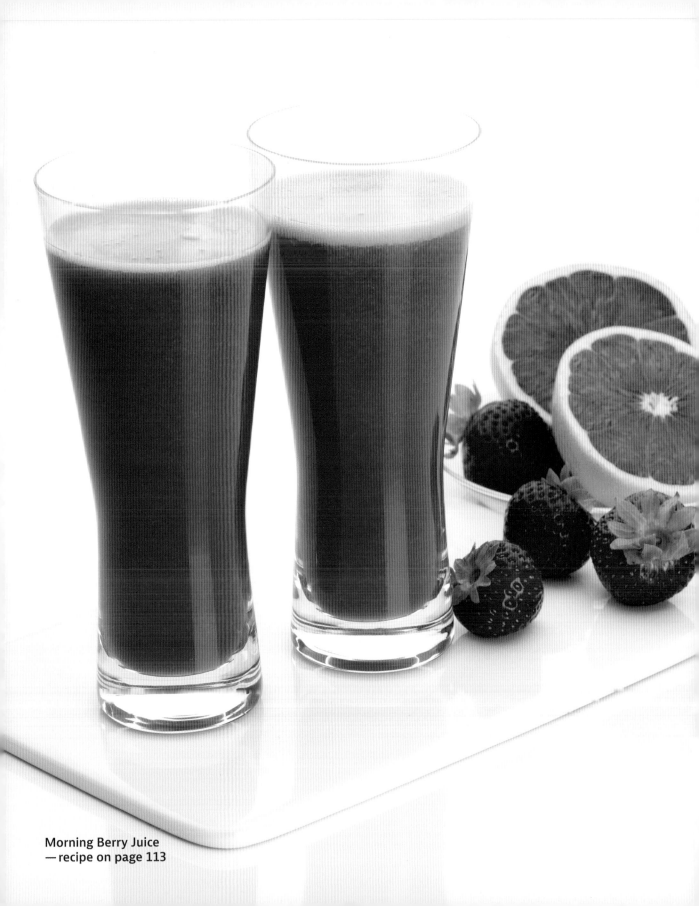

Morning Berry Juice
— recipe on page 113

Juicer Recipes

Sweet

Savory

Carrot Berry Gulp

Calories	154
Fat	1 g
Sat fat	0
Protein	3 g
Carbohydrate	36 g
Fiber	10 g

The double punch of both strawberries and blackberries gives you the antioxidants to stave off oxidative attacks, and recent research shows that berry consumption may protect against Alzheimer's disease. Beta-carotene from the carrots and vitamin C and citrus phytochemicals just add to the firepower. Just about any berry can substitute for another, although dark-colored berries, such as blueberries and blackberries, will alter the color of the juice.

🫐	1 cup (250 mL)	blackberries (4½ oz/128 grams)
🍓	1½ cups (375 mL)	hulled whole strawberries (9 oz/245 grams)
🍊	1	peeled large (9½ oz/270 grams) navel orange
🥕	2	medium carrots (3½ oz/105 grams)

1. Wash all produce well. Use a produce brush to clean carrots.

2. Place into juicer in order listed and juice.

Makes 2 servings (2 cups/500 mL/450 g)

Phytochemicals
Alpha- and beta-carotene, chlorogenic acid, ellagic acid, ferulic acid, gallic acid, kaempferol, lutein, luteolin, lycopene, pelargonidin, matairesinol, secoisolariciresinol, zeaxanthin

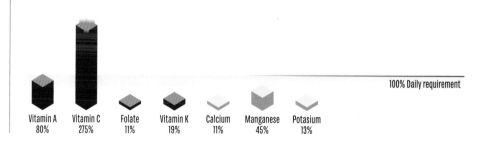

| Vitamin A 80% | Vitamin C 275% | Folate 11% | Vitamin K 19% | Calcium 11% | Manganese 45% | Potasium 13% | 100% Daily requirement |

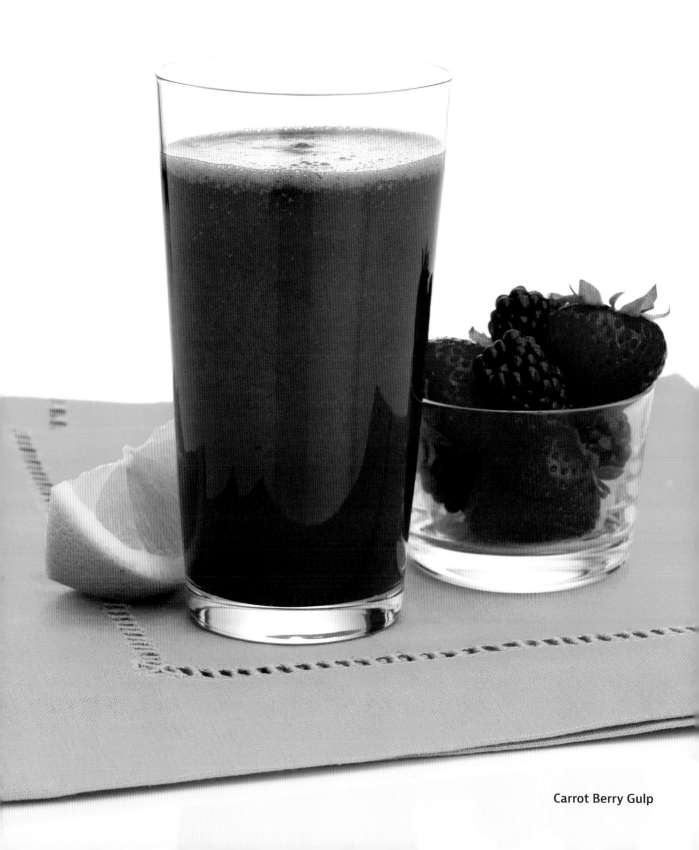

Carrot Berry Gulp

Smooth Kaling

Calories	191
Fat	0
Sat fat	0
Protein	3 g
Carbohydrate	36 g
Fiber	8 g

Super Enhancer Tip

Try stirring in some cinnamon. Go lightly at first, then see if you can build up to at least ½ tsp (2 mL) when you are familiar with the mix of flavors.

A common misconception is that only brightly colored fruits and vegetables contain healthy phytochemicals, since many of these compounds are bright pigments. The honeydew melon, however, dispels that myth with a healthy dose of antioxidants. The same is true for the apple, with scientific papers describing the numerous phytochemicals in this favorite. And, of course, kale and carrots are both hard to beat for essential nutrients and phytochemicals. That combination is the reason that one serving of this delicious juice provides four times the DRI for vitamin A.

	1½ cups (375 mL)	peeled seeded honeydew melon (15 oz/425 g)
	3	medium carrots (6½ oz/190 g)
	3 cups (750 mL)	packed chopped kale (2 oz/60 g)
	1	cored large Fuji apple (7½ oz/215 g)

1. Wash all produce well. Use a produce brush to scrub carrots.

2. Place ingredients into juicer in order listed and juice.

Makes 2 servings (2½ cups/525 mL/585 g)

Phytochemicals

Alpha- and beta carotene, catechins, hydroxycinnamic acids (caffeic acid, ferulic acid), indole-3-carbinol, lycopene, luteolin, lutein, procyanidins, quercetin, secoisolariciresinol, ursolic acid, zeaxanthin

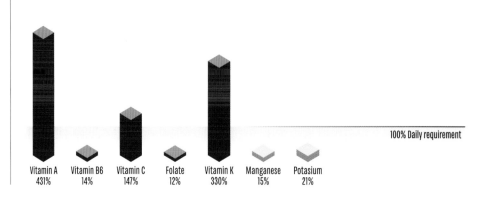

Vitamin A	Vitamin B6	Vitamin C	Folate	Vitamin K	Manganese	Potasium
431%	14%	147%	12%	330%	15%	21%

100% Daily requirement

Gingered Mango

This recipe is an example of using superfoods that you wouldn't normally think of putting together. Most people don't think that combining garlic and ginger would work for the average palate. However, the highly aromatic flavor of mango and the acidity of the orange make for great cover! The mango contains several phytochemicals unique to it, as does ginger, which has been a medicinal plant from ancient times. A more adventurous person can increase the amount of garlic to 3 cloves to obtain even more health benefits.

Calories		204
Fat		0
Sat fat		0
Protein		4 g
Carbohydrate		50 g
Fiber		8 g

	1	peeled medium orange (10 oz/280 g)
	1 piece (1 inch/2.5 cm)	gingerroot (¼ oz/6 g)
	1 clove	garlic
	1	pitted medium mango (9 oz/260 g)
	3	medium carrots (8 oz/230 g)

1. Wash all produce well. Peel ginger; use a produce brush to clean carrots.

2. Place ingredients into juicer in order listed and juice.

Makes 2 servings (1¾ cups/475 mL/430 g)

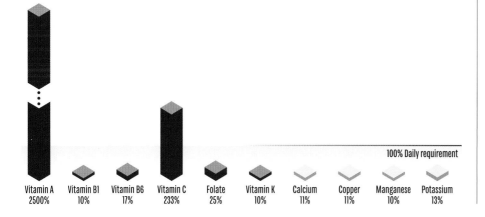

Vitamin A	Vitamin B1	Vitamin B6	Vitamin C	Folate	Vitamin K	Calcium	Copper	Manganese	Potassium
2500%	10%	17%	233%	25%	10%	11%	11%	10%	13%

100% Daily requirement

Phytochemicals
Allicin, anacardic acid, beta-carotene, caffeic acid, catechins, coumarin, cryptoxanthin, diallyl sulfide, ferulic acid, gallic acid, gingerole, kaempferol, limonene, lutein, luteolin, lycopene, mangiferin, oleanolic acid, phytoene, phytofluene, quercetin, secoisolariciresinol, tannins, zeaxanthin

Fruit vs Veggie

Calories	123
Fat	0
Sat fat	0
Protein	2 g
Carbohydrate	29 g
Fiber	6 g

Super Enhancer Tip

This juice is low in calories. To boost the protein without adding too many extra calories, consider adding a tablespoon of whey protein. Just 1 tbsp (15 mL) of most powdered whey products adds 5 grams of high-quality protein for just 25 calories.

Several ingredients in this juice contain one of the most potent antioxidants, lycopene. In addition, for only 123 calories, you'll get more than twice the DRI for vitamin C, another key antioxidant — how's that for nutrient dense? Any apple can be substituted for the Red Delicious variety, but it is one of the sweeter apples, which helps to blend with the garlic.

	2	medium plum (Roma) tomatoes (4 oz/125 g)
	1	seeded ribbed medium red bell pepper (4 oz/120 g)
	1 clove	garlic
	1 cup	packed baby spinach (1¼ oz/33 g)
	½ cup (125 mL)	hulled strawberries (4 oz/115 g)
	1	cored medium Red Delicious apple (7½ oz/215 g)

1. Wash all produce well.

2. Place ingredients into juicer in order listed and juice.

Makes 2 servings (2 cups/500 mL/490 g)

Phytochemicals

Alpha- and beta-carotene, allicin, catechins, chlorogenic acid, chlorophyll, coumestrol, cryptoxanthin, diallyl sulfide, ellagic acid, gallic acid, hydroxycinnamic acids (caffeic acid, ferulic acid), kaempferol, limonene, lycopene, matairesinol, oleanolic acid, pelargonidin, procyanidins, quercetin, secoisolariciresinol, ursolic acid, zeaxanthin

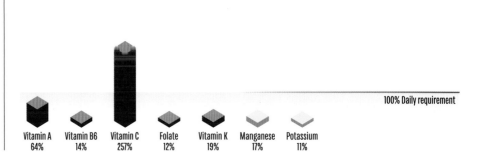

Vitamin A 64%	Vitamin B6 14%	Vitamin C 257%	Folate 12%	Vitamin K 19%	Manganese 17%	Potassium 11%	100% Daily requirement

Blackberry Citrus

The impressive array of phytochemicals in this juice, and the fantastic blend of fruit flavors, make it a perfect breakfast treat. Along with other berries, blackberries are one of the fruits highest in antioxidants and may help prevent cognitive decline as we age. The orange and lime add the special phytochemicals found exclusively in citrus fruits.

1		peeled medium orange (9½ oz/260 g)
1		cored medium Fuji apple (7 oz/190 g)
¼		peeled medium lime (1 oz/30 g)
1 cup (250 mL)		blackberries (7 oz/190 g)

1. Wash all produce well.

2. Place ingredients into juicer in order listed and juice.

Makes 2 servings (1¾ cups/425 mL/410 g)

Calories	159
Fat	0
Sat fat	0
Protein	2 g
Carbohydrate	39 g
Fiber	10 g

Super Enhancer Tip

This juice is low in calories, so the addition of chia seeds or a mixture of seeds will provide the perfect addition of protein, fiber and more phytochemicals. Adding ½ tbsp (7 mL) of seed mixture adds 3 grams of fiber and protein for just 40 calories.

Phytochemicals
Catechins, coumarin, cryptoxanthin, cyanidin, ellagic acid, ferulic acid, hydroxycinnamic acids (caffeic acid, ferulic acid), lignans, limonene, lutein, phenolic acids, phytoene, phytofluene, procyanidins, quercetin, stilbenoids, tannins, ursolic acid, zeaxanthin

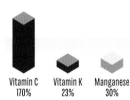

100% Daily requirement

Vitamin C 170%   Vitamin K 23%   Manganese 30%

Carrot Limeberry

Calories	160
Fat	1 g
Sat fat	0
Protein	4 g
Carbohydrate	38 g
Fiber	13 g

Super Enhancer Tip

Adding a protein base like tofu or yogurt makes this delicious juice a more substantial meal replacement. Talk about a power lunch — whisk in 1 slice (3 oz/85 g) of silken tofu, which blends easily. You'll add 6 grams of protein and important phytochemicals, isoflavones.

Phytochemicals

Alpha- and beta-carotene, anthocyanidins, ellagic acid, lignans, luteolin, lycopene, hesperidin, isolimonexic acid, limonexic acid, limonene, neohesperidin, pelargonidin, phenolic acids, quercetin, rutin, secoisolariciresinol, stilbenoids, tannins

With just a few ingredients, this recipe knocks it out of the park for both taste and nutrition. Check the vitamin A content at seven times the DRI. Like all berries, the antioxidant phytochemicals in raspberries are especially high. Recent studies using raspberry extract reported blood-pressure-lowering effects and inhibition of leukemia cells. This juice will be a great way to greet the day!

	5	medium carrots (7 oz/210 g)
	¼	peeled medium lime (1 oz/30 g)
	1 cup (250 mL)	raspberries (3½ oz/110 g)

1. Wash all produce well. Scrub carrots with a produce brush.

2. Place ingredients into juicer in order listed and juice.

Makes 1 serving (1 cup/250 mL/225 g)

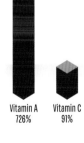

Vitamin A	Vitamin C	Vitamin K	Manganese
726%	91%	11%	37%

100% Daily requirement

Gingered Pearberry

Ginger adds flavor and potent phytochemicals to this interesting blend of fruits and carrots. Studies have shown that one of these phytochemicals, DGE, was not only an effective antioxidant, it also inhibited the growth of breast cancer cells. From a nutritional standpoint, different pear varieties are similar. However, the flavors can be quite different, so try substituting your favorite for the Bosc pear.

	1 piece (2 inches/5 cm)	gingerroot (½ oz/12 g)
	1 cup (250 mL)	blackberries (6½ oz/185 g)
	1	cored medium Bosc pear (7 oz/200 g)
	3	medium carrots (7 oz/200 g)

1. Wash all produce well. Peel ginger, leave skin on pear and scrub carrots with a produce brush.

2. Place ingredients into juicer in order listed and juice.

Makes 2 servings (1½ cups/375 mL/320 g)

Calories	145
Fat	1 g
Sat fat	0
Protein	3 g
Carbohydrate	35 g
Fiber	10 g

Super Enhancer Tip

The yield is less than 1 cup (250 ml) per serving, so to increase volume, try adding ⅓ cup (75 mL) coconut water. This will only add 15 calories, but it will further boost the antioxidants in this tasty juice.

Vitamin A	Vitamin C	Vitamin K	Copper	Manganese		100% Daily requirement
365%	50%	27%	12%	31%		

Phytochemicals
Alpha- and beta-carotene, anthocyanidins, caffeic acid, chlorogenic acid, cyanidin, 6-dehydrogingerdione (DGE), ellagic acid, gingersole, lignans, limonene, lutein, luteolin, lycopene, phenolic acids, secoisolariciresinol, shogaols, stilbenoids, tannins

Tropical Kale

Calories	214
Fat	1
Sat fat	0
Protein	4 g
Carbohydrate	53 g
Fiber	6 g

Super Enhancer Tip

Turn this powerful juice into a meal replacement for later in the day, when most people eat more of their calories. Stir in Greek yogurt for a more pudding-like consistency, and you've got a great-tasting dessert. Or to reclaim some of the fiber and also add protein, stir in 1 tbsp (15 mL) of chia seeds for an additional 5 grams of fiber and 3 grams of protein.

Phytochemicals

Alpha- and beta-carotene, anacardic acid, caffeic acid, catechins, chlorogenic acid, chlorophyll, cryptoxanthin, ferulic acid, gallic acid, indole-3-carbinol, kaempferol, lutein, mangiferin, quercetin, tannins, zeaxanthin

It's a bit higher in calories, but this high-powered recipe is loaded with essential vitamins and minerals. All the ingredients are nutrition stars by themselves, and the combination is even more nutritious, with a taste that's hard to describe. A recent study showed that eating kiwi every day significantly lowered blood pressure.

	¼	peeled cored medium pineapple (9 oz/260 g)
	1¾ cups (425 mL)	pitted mango (10 oz/290 grams)
	2	medium kiwifruit (7 oz/190 g)
	4 cups (1 L)	packed chopped kale (2 oz/55 g)

1. Wash all produce well, but you don't need to peel the mango or kiwi.

2. Place ingredients into juicer in order listed and juice.

Makes 2 servings (2 cups/500 mL/410 g)

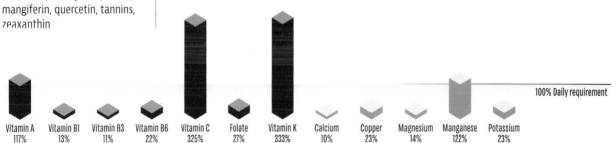

| Vitamin A 117% | Vitamin B1 13% | Vitamin B3 11% | Vitamin B6 22% | Vitamin C 325% | Folate 27% | Vitamin K 333% | Calcium 10% | Copper 23% | Magnesium 14% | Manganese 122% | Potassium 23% |

100% Daily requirement

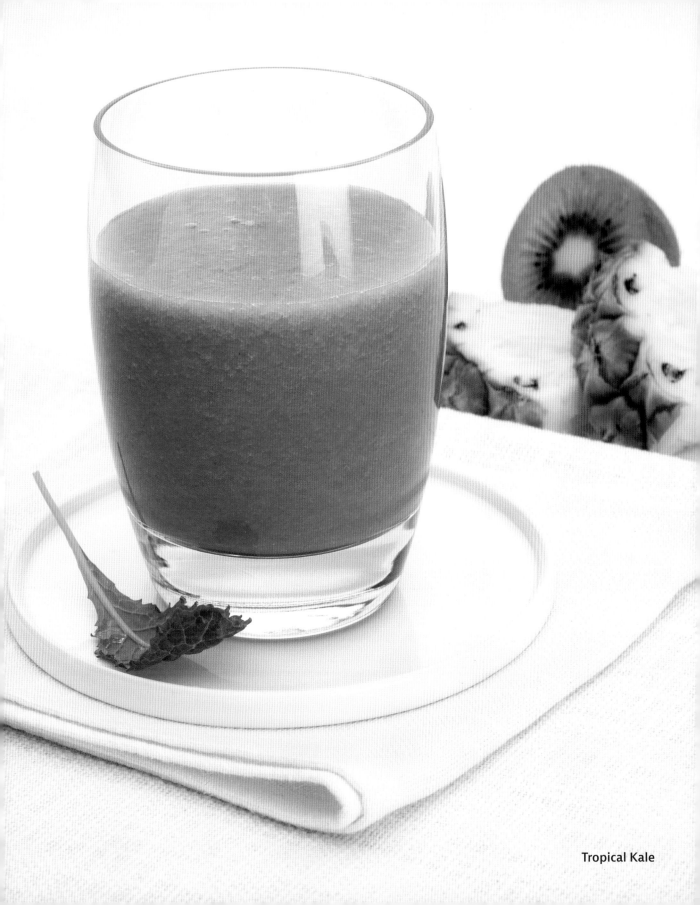

Tropical Kale

Berried Island Treasure

Calories	250
Fat	1 g
Sat fat	0
Protein	5 g
Carbohydrate	64 g
Fiber	5 g

The carrot and the kale double up on carotenoids, providing a diverse mix and high content of antioxidants. The pineapple adds sweetness and a zingy flavor, rounded out by raspberries for additional sweetness and even more phytochemicals.

	¼	peeled cored medium pineapple (10 oz/300 g)
	2 cups (500 mL)	packed chopped kale (1 oz/33 g)
	1½ cups (375 mL)	raspberries (2 oz/60 g)
	2	medium carrots (5½ oz/160 g)

1. Wash all produce well. Scrub carrots with a produce brush.

2. Place ingredients into juicer in order listed and juice.

Makes 1 serving (1 cup/250 mL/255 g)

Phytochemicals
Alpha- and beta-carotene, anthocyanidins, caffeic acid, chlorogenic acid, cyanidin, 6-dehydrogingerdione (DGE), ellagic acid, gingersole, lignans, limonene, lutein, luteolin, lycopene, phenolic acids, secoisolariciresinol, shogaols, stilbenoids, tannins

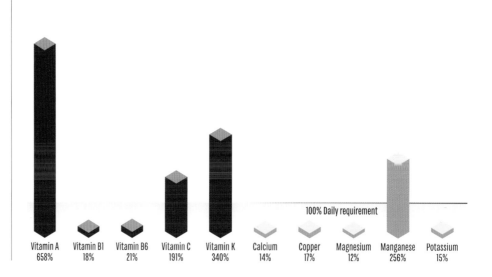

Vitamin A 658%	Vitamin B1 18%	Vitamin B6 21%	Vitamin C 191%	Vitamin K 340%	Calcium 14%	Copper 17%	Magnesium 12%	Manganese 256%	Potassium 15%

100% Daily requirement

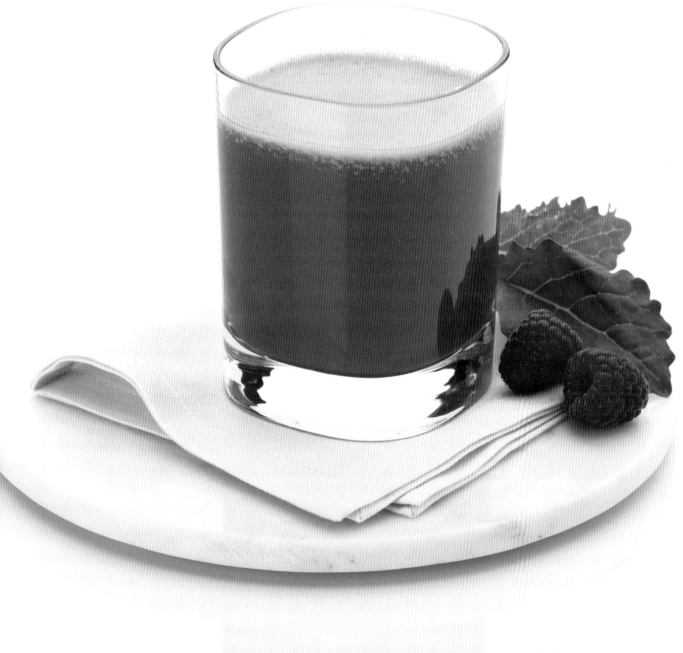

Berried Island Treasure

Berried Grapes

Calories	157
Fat	1 g
Sat fat	0
Protein	3 g
Carbohydrate	40 g
Fiber	5 g

The double dose of berries provides both tartness and sweet flavor to this recipe, along with antioxidants to fight dementia. Ginger adds flavor and phytochemicals, and if you like the taste, you may want to add more. As well, recent research has pointed to a possible mechanism for the grape's phytochemical, resveratrol, in slowing the aging process.

- 2 cups (500 mL) black seedless grapes (13½ oz/380 g)

  1 piece (1 inch/2.5 cm) gingerroot (½ oz/12 g)

- ½ cup (125 mL) blackberries (3 oz/88 g)

- 1 cup (250 ml) hulled strawberries (6 oz/160 g)

1. Wash all produce well and peel ginger.

2. Place ingredients into juicer in order listed and juice.

Makes 2 servings (1¾ cups /425 mL/380 g)

Phytochemicals
Catechins,chlorogenic acid, cyanidin, ellagic acid, gallic acid, gingerol, 6 dehydrogingerdione (DGE) kaempferol, lignans, limonene, matairesinol, pelargonidin, phenolic acids, piceatannol, pterostilbene, resveratrol, secoisolariciresinol, shogaols, stilbenoids, tannins, tartaric acid, zeaxanthin

100% Daily requirement

Vitamin C	Vitamin K	Copper	Manganese	Potassium
24%	39%	14%	20%	11%

Mango Carotene

The vibrant orange of both mango and carrot indicate the presence of several carotenoids and plenty of vitamin A. You can substitute any green for the kale, although not all greens will give you the indole-3-carbinol, which has cancer-fighting properties.

- 5 medium carrots (12 oz/340 g)
- 2 cups (500 mL) packed chopped kale (1 oz/30 g)
- 1 medium pitted mango (11 oz/320 g)

1. Wash all produce well. Scrub carrots with produce brush; leave skin on mango.

2. Place ingredients into juicer in order listed and juice.

Makes 1 serving (1¼ cups/300 mL/285 g)

Calories	359
Fat	1 g
Sat fat	0
Protein	8 g
Carbohydrate	86 g
Fiber	14 g

Super Enhancer Tips

Try adding a dash of cinnamon to the juice for additional health benefits and taste.

This recipe is high calorie for the low volume, but it does contain protein. To boost the protein without adding many calories and use as a meal replacement, try stirring in some spirulina powder. Just 2 tsp (10 mL) of most brands will add 4 grams of protein and more vitamin A and antioxidants.

Phytochemicals
Alpha- and beta-carotene, anacardic acid, caffeic acid, catechins, cryptoxanthin, gallic acid, indole-3-carbinol, kaempferol, lutein, luteolin, lycopene, mangiferin, quercetin, secoisolariciresinol, tannins, zeaxanthin

100% Daily requirement

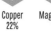

Vitamin A	Vitamin B3	Vitamin B6	Vitamin C	Folate	Vitamin K	Calcium	Copper	Magnesium	Manganese	Potassium
1,335%	12%	23%	296%	37%	313%	16%	22%	11%	21%	19%

Tartberry Pear

Calories	206
Fat	1 g
Sat fat	0
Protein	3 g
Carbohydrate	54 g
Fiber	9 g

A hint of lime livens up this delicious blend of favorite fruits. The grape provides resveratrol, the anti-aging phytochemical, while the strawberries have excited health enthusiasts by lowering the risk for cognitive decline associated with aging. The d'Anjou pear, which derives its name from a cultivar originating in either France or Belgium, consists of several varieties. The pear in this recipe is the green d'Anjou, which does not change color as it ripens.

🍇	1 cup (250 mL)	black seedless grapes (6 oz/170 g)
🍓	1 cup (250 mL)	hulled strawberries (6 oz/160 grams)
🍐	2	cored medium d'Anjou pears (14 oz/400 g)
🍋	½	peeled medium lime (1¼ oz/36 g)

1. Wash all produce well.

2. Place ingredients into juicer in order listed and juice.

Makes 2 servings (1½ cups/375 mL/295 g)

Phytochemicals
ALA, Anthocyanidins, caffeic acid, catechin, catechol, chlorogenic acid, cyanidin, ellagic acid, friedelin, gallic acid, kaempferol, lutein, matairesinol, pelargonidin, piceatannol, phytosterols, pterostilbene, resveratrol, secoisolariciresinol, tartaric acid, ursolic acid, zeaxanthin

100% Daily requirement

Vitamin C	Vitamin K	Copper	Potassium
28%	26%	13%	12%

Berry Beany Citrus

The vegetables outweigh the fruit in this recipe, but you wouldn't know it by the sweet and tart taste. Among the many phytochemicals, squalene brings antioxidant, antibacterial, anticancer and immune-enhancing effects. This juice also gives you twice the recommended level of vitamin A for the entire day. Since it's in the form of carotenoids, precursor compounds for active vitamin A, the body only converts the amount it needs. The remaining carotenoids act as antioxidants to fight free radicals.

Calories	147
Fat	1 g
Sat fat	0
Protein	5 g
Carbohydrate	34 g
Fiber	10 g

	⅓ cup (75 mL)	green beans (6 oz/170 g)
	1	medium tomato (9½ oz/270 g)
	1 cup (250 mL)	baby carrots (4 oz/115 g)
	1	peeled medium orange (7 oz/195 g)
	¾ cup (175 mL)	raspberries (3½ oz/100 g)

1. Wash all produce well.

2. Place ingredients into juicer in order listed and juice.

Makes 2 servings (2 cups/500 mL/440 g)

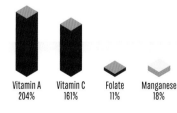

Vitamin A 204%   Vitamin C 161%   Folate 11%   Manganese 18%

100% Daily requirement

Phytochemicals
ALA, alpha- and beta-carotene, anthocyanidins, bergapten, caffeic acid, campesterol, chlorogenic acid, chlorophyll, coumarin, cryptoxanthin, ellagic acid, eugenol, ferulic acid, genistein, geraniol, inositol, limonene, lupeol, lutein, luteolin, lycopene, naringenin, pelargonidin, phytoene, phytofluene, phytosterols, quercetin, rutin, secoisolariciresinol, squalene, trigonelline, zeaxanthin

A Date with Chocolate

Calories	50
Fat	3 g
Sat fat	0
Protein	2 g
Carbohydrate	5 g
Fiber	1 g

This simple ganache is a great dessert for chocolate lovers with their eyes on health. It features almond butter, which not only provides a great mouth feel but also heart-healthy fats, manganese and vitamin E. You can easily make your own almond butter (see step 2 below) or you can purchase it at most stores. The dates are another superfood, providing vitamins, minerals, fiber and phytochemicals, and, of course, a wonderful sweet taste. The final touch is cocoa, which boosts the antioxidants to an almost unprecedented level.

1 cup (250 mL)	pitted Medjool dates (10 to 12)
2 cups (500 ml)	water
1 cup (250 mL)	almonds or store-bought almond butter (roasted and unsalted works best if making your own)
1 cup (250 mL)	unsweetened cocoa powder
1 tbsp (15 ml)	pure vanilla extract

1. Soak dates in water for 2 hours, then drain but save the soaking water.

2. To make almond butter, feed nuts in slowly, a few at a time. You will need to process the butter more than once until the desired consistency is achieved. With successive runs, use plunger. Roasted nuts work better than raw, but each will provide a different flavor.

3. Transfer dates to a blender or food processor. Add almond butter, cocoa powder, vanilla and 1 cup soaking liquid. Cover and blend until smooth and creamy, adding more water, approximately ½ cup (125 mL) at a time, until the desired consistency is achieved, about 2 minutes. In a dessert bowl or plate, serve the chocolate ganache over diced cooked apples or strawberries.

Makes 3½ cups (825 mL), about 50 servings (1 tbsp/15 mL each)

Phytochemicals
ALA, beta-carotene, beta-sitosterol, caffeic acid, catechins, chlorogenic acid, chlorophyll, coumarin, cyanidins, ferulic acid, gallic acid, flavonols, lutein, lycopene, oleic acid, phytosterols, pipecolic acid, polyphenols, proanthocyanidins, tannins, trigonelline

Vitamins and minerals: None present at 10% level

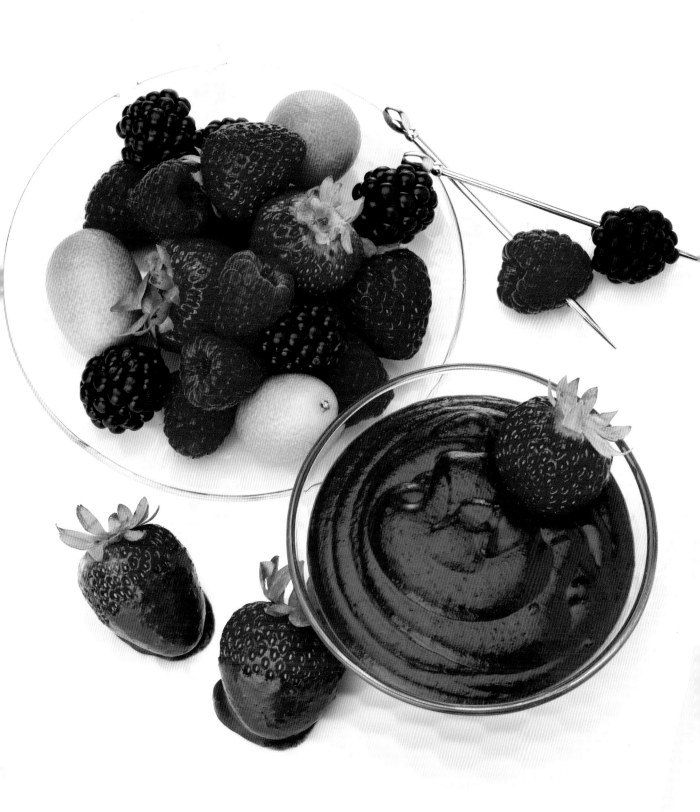

A Date with Chocolate

Duck Duck Gooseberry

Calories	175
Fat	1 g
Sat fat	0
Protein	2 g
Carbohydrate	41 g
Fiber	6 g

Super Enhancer Tips

Add 1 tbsp (15 mL) milled flax for protein, fiber and ALA.

Add 1 tbsp (15 mL) seed mixture for the above, plus numerous phytochemicals and prebiotics.

The kiwi, also called a Chinese gooseberry, provides an incredible 26% of the daily need for iron and three times the recommended level for vitamin C. This recipe makes a super breakfast, and you can add some flax and seed mixture to put back some of the fiber, along with more phytochemicals and protein.

	3	medium kiwifruit (9 oz/240 g)
	1 cup (250 mL)	black seedless grapes (6 oz/165 g)
	½ cup (125 mL)	baby carrots (2 oz/55 g)

1. Wash kiwi (don't peel) and grapes.

2. Place ingredients into juicer in order listed and juice.

Makes 2 servings (2 cups/500 mL/460 g)

Phytochemicals
Alpha- and beta-carotene, bergapten, caffeic acid, campesterol, catechins, chlorogenic acid, coumarin, cryptoxanthin, cyanidin, ellagic acid, ferulic acid, geraniol, lupeol, lutein, luteolin, lycopene, phytofluene, phytosterols, piceatannol, pterostilbene, resveratrol, secoisolariciresinol, tartaric acid, zeaxanthin

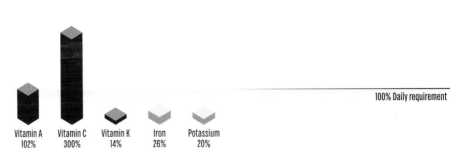

100% Daily requirement

Vitamin A	Vitamin C	Vitamin K	Iron	Potassium
102%	300%	14%	26%	20%

Morning Berry Juice

With only three ingredients, this sweet, citrus-based juice is quick, easy and incredibly delicious. Its impressive nutrient profile also makes it a perfect meal replacement with the addition of protein and fiber. For a creamy taste, add vanilla whey protein powder and pick up some fiber with seed mixture. With the extra protein and fiber, it will keep you satisfied until lunch.

Calories		207
Fat		1 g
Sat fat		0
Protein		4 g
Carbohydrate		53 g
Fiber		8 g

🍊	1	peeled medium red or pink grapefruit (13 oz/360 g)
🍓	1 cup (250 mL)	hulled strawberries (6 oz/150 g)
🥕	½ cup (125 mL)	baby carrots (2 oz/58 g)

1. Wash strawberries.

2. Place ingredients into juicer in order listed and juice.

Makes 1 serving (1½ cups/375 mL/350 g)

Super Enhancer Tips

👍 Add 1 tbsp (15 mL) vanilla whey protein powder for extra protein.

👍 Add 1 tbsp (15 mL) seed mixture for protein, fiber and prebiotics.

Phytochemicals

ALA, alpha- and beta-carotene, bergapten, caffeic acid, campesterol, , catechin, catechol, chlorogenic acid, coumarin, cryptoxanthin, ellagic acid, ferulic acid, gallic acid, geraniol, hesperetin, hesperidin, isorhamnetin, kaempferol, limonene, lupeol, lutein, luteolin, lycopene, matairesinol, pelargonidin, phytoene, phytofluene, phytosterols, quercetin, secoisolariciresinol, zeaxanthin

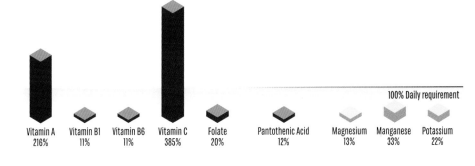

| Vitamin A 216% | Vitamin B1 11% | Vitamin B6 11% | Vitamin C 385% | Folate 20% | Pantothenic Acid 12% | Magnesium 13% | Manganese 33% | Potassium 22% |

100% Daily requirement

Can't Beet It

Calories	167
Fat	1 g
Sat fat	0
Protein	4 g
Carbohydrate	41 g
Fiber	9 g

Both the parsnip and the beet contain interesting phytochemicals. The beet contains betaine, which protects the heart. The parsnip contains bergapten, which has anti-inflammatory and anticlotting effects, both of which also protect the heart. When juicing these roots, however, it's important to remember that both impart a sharp flavor. The parsnip has a particularly noticeable taste that is reminiscent of cinnamon. When using these roots, be sure to include a fruit that is extra sweet and also provides a bit of cover, as does the orange. The combination of these three ingredients is perfectly balanced to bring out just a touch of the interesting root flavors. They also balance perfectly from a nutritional standpoint, with the orange providing the nutrients that the roots don't contain.

	1	beet (3½ oz/100 g)
	⅓ cup (75 mL)	parsnip (1½ oz/44 g)
	1	peeled large orange (6½ oz/185 g)

1. Wash all produce well. Use a vegetable brush to scrub beet and parsnip; chop off top and bottom of beet and peel parsnip.

2. Place ingredients into juicer in order listed and juice.

Makes 1 serving (1¼ cups/300 ml/330 g)

Phytochemicals
ALA, alpha- and beta-carotene, bergapten, betaine, camphene, coumarin, cryptoxanthin, ferulic acid, limonene, lutein, myristicin, phytoene, phytofluene, phytosterols, tartaric acid, zeaxanthin

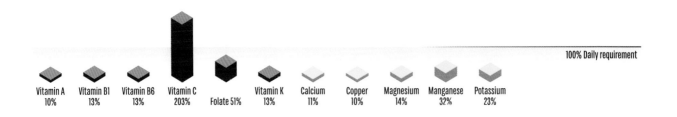

Vitamin A	Vitamin B1	Vitamin B6	Vitamin C	Folate	Vitamin K	Calcium	Copper	Magnesium	Manganese	Potassium	100% Daily requirement
10%	13%	13%	203%	51%	13%	11%	10%	14%	32%	23%	

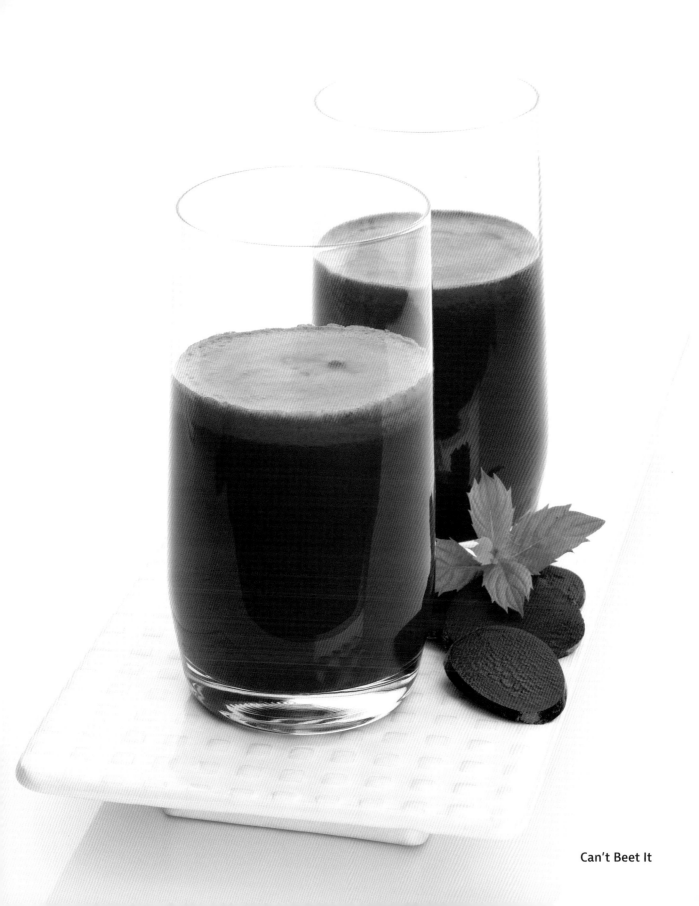

Can't Beet It

Pearberry Cress

Calories	163
Fat	1 g
Sat fat	0
Protein	5 g
Carbohydrate	38 g
Fiber	16 g

This recipe combines the sweetness and tartness of the pear and raspberry, while including a high-powered green, watercress. A study reported that watercress combated compounds that cause inflammation and cancer. And those effects related to phytochemicals, but watercress is also loaded with essential nutrients.

	3 cups (750 mL)	packed watercress (3½ oz/100 g)
	½	cored large Bosc pear (3½ oz/95 g)
	1½ cups (275 mL)	raspberries (6½ oz/185 g)

1. Wash all produce well. Chop off excess stems from watercress.

2. Place ingredients into juicer in order listed and juice.

Makes 1 serving (1½ cups/375 mL/380 g)

Phytochemicals
ALA, anthocyanidins, beta-carotene, caffeic acid, chlorogenic acid, cyanidin, ellagic acid, friedelin, lutein, pelargonidin, phytosterols, quercetin, ursolic acid

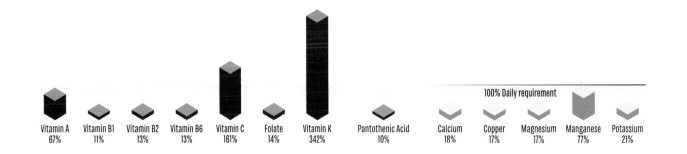

| Vitamin A 67% | Vitamin B1 11% | Vitamin B2 13% | Vitamin B6 13% | Vitamin C 161% | Folate 14% | Vitamin K 342% | Pantothenic Acid 10% | Calcium 18% | Copper 17% | Magnesium 17% | Manganese 77% | Potassium 21% |

100% Daily requirement

Three-Orange Zucchini

The tiny kumquat is not familiar to many people, but it's worth getting to know. The entire fruit is edible, so it's perfect for juicing. It is nutrient dense, with both essential nutrients and phytochemicals for not many calories. The zucchini in this recipe is baby zucchini, which is much nicer than regular zucchini because the skin is thin and tender. If you grow zucchini in the summer, however, this is a great way to use it.

Calories	263
Fat	1 g
Sat fat	0
Protein	8 g
Carbohydrate	60 g
Fiber	17 g

🍓	½ cup (125 mL)	hulled strawberries (3 oz/80 g)
🥒	1	baby zucchini (3½ oz/100 g)
🫐	6	kumquats (approx. 4 oz/115 g each)
🍊	½	peeled large orange (5 oz/140 g)
🥕	2	medium carrots (5 oz/140 g)

1. Wash all produce well. Use a vegetable brush to scrub carrots.

2. Place ingredients into juicer in order listed and juice.

Makes 1 serving (1 cup/250 mL/222 g)

Phytochemicals
Alpha- and beta-carotene, bergapten,beta-sitosterol, caffeic acid, campesterol, catechin, catechol, chlorogenic acid, coumarin, cryptoxanthin, cucurbitacin, ellagic acid, ferulic acid, gallic acid, geraniol, hespertin, isoflavones,kaempferol, limonene, limonin, lupeol, lutein, luteolin, lycopene, matairesinol, pelargonidin, phytoene,phytofluene, phytosterols, secoisolariciresinol, zeaxanthin

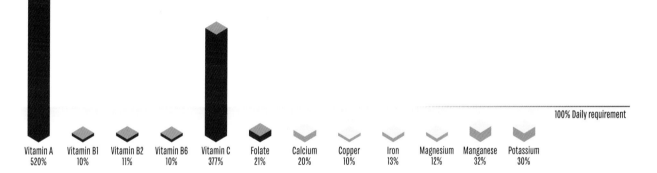

Vitamin A	Vitamin B1	Vitamin B2	Vitamin B6	Vitamin C	Folate	Calcium	Copper	Iron	Magnesium	Manganese	Potassium
520%	10%	11%	10%	377%	21%	20%	10%	13%	12%	32%	30%

100% Daily requirement

Pomberry Cress

Calories	185
Fat	2 g
Sat fat	0
Protein	5 g
Carbohydrate	42 g
Fiber	25 g

Phytochemicals
Beta-carotene, caffeic acid, catechin, catechol, chlorogenic acid, cyanidin, ellagic acid, gallic acid, kaempferol, lutein, matairesinol, pelargonidin, phytosterols, punicalagins,sec oisolariciresinol, urosolic acid, zeaxanthin

The pomegranate, which hails from ancient Persia, has steadily grown in popularity ever since its deep burgundy juice hit the markets a decade ago. Since then, prepackaged seeds have also become available due to consumer demand for this superfood. A recent clinical trial showed that pomegranate extract reduced prostate-specific antigen (PSA) levels, an indication of disease progression, in prostate cancer patients. The peel is too bitter to consume or use intact in a juicer. However, removing the peel and leaving the membranes holding the seeds is adequate with a juicer. For blender recipes, it's best to choose the prepackaged seeds.

🍓	1 cup (250 mL)	hulled strawberries (6 oz/150 g)
🟤	½	peeled medium pomegranate (6 ½ oz/160 grams))
🌿	1 cup (250 mL)	packed watercress (1¼ oz/35 g)

1. Wash all produce well. Chop excess stems from watercress.

2. Place ingredients into juicer in order listed and juice.

Makes 1 serving (¾ cup /175 mL/175 g)

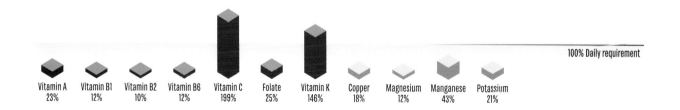

	100% Daily requirement

Vitamin A	Vitamin B1	Vitamin B2	Vitamin B6	Vitamin C	Folate	Vitamin K	Copper	Magnesium	Manganese	Potassium
23%	12%	10%	12%	199%	25%	146%	18%	12%	43%	21%

Pomagrapple

This recipe blends three fruits in a delightful juice to start your day. The Braeburn is a tart apple and you can easily substitute any other variety, since the pomegranate also provides tartness. In many countries, particularly in the Middle East, the juice from the pomegranate is made into syrup, or molasses, that is used as an ingredient in many dishes. To make pomegranate syrup, add 2 cups (500 mL) of pomegranate juice to ½ cup (125 mL) sugar and ½ tbsp (7 ml) freshly squeezed lemon juice. Heat the mixture on medium heat, stirring occasionally. When the sugar is dissolved, reduce heat one notch and continue simmering until the volume has reduced by about half, or about 40 minutes. The syrup is an excellent addition to sautéed leafy green vegetables, such as kale.

🍎	1	cored medium Braeburn apple (6 oz/160 g)
🟤	⅓	peeled medium pomegranate (3½ oz/100 g)
🍇	½ cup (125 mL)	red seedless grapes (2½ oz/70 g)

1. Wash all produce well.

2. Place ingredients into juicer in order listed and juice.

Makes 1 serving (1 cup/250 mL/205 g)

Calories	215
Fat	1 g
Sat fat	0
Protein	2 g
Carbohydrate	57 g
Fiber	9 g

Super Enhancer Tip

👍 Stir in a tablespoon (15 mL) of seed mix to add prebiotic fiber, protein and additional phytochemicals.

100% Daily requirement

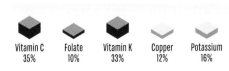

Vitamin C 35% Folate 10% Vitamin K 33% Copper 12% Potassium 16%

Phytochemicals
Catechins, caffeic acid, chlorogenic acid, cyanidin, ellagic acid, ferulic acid, isorhamnetin, phytosterols, pic eatannol, procyanidins, pterost ilbene, punicalagins, quercetin, resveratrol, tartaric acid, ursolic acid

Star-Cressed Lovers

Calories	159
Fat	0
Sat fat	0
Protein	3 g
Carbohydrate	41 g
Fiber	7 g

Although any apple can be substituted for the Fuji, this variety has a nice blend of tartness and sweetness. It gets its name from the town in Japan where the hybrid was developed. Like all apples, it contains numerous phytochemicals, enough so that scientific papers have been written entirely on this subject. The orange provides several essential nutrients the apple doesn't contain, especially vitamin C and the B vitamin folate. Both of these fruits blend well with the watercress, which brings more antioxidants to this delicious juice.

	1 cup (250 mL)	packed watercress (1¼ oz/35 g)
	½	cored medium Fuji apple (3 oz/90 g)
	1	peeled small orange (8 oz/220 g)

1. Wash all produce well. Chop excess stems from watercress.

2. Place ingredients into juicer in order listed and juice.

Makes 1 serving (1 cup/250 mL/240 g)

Phytochemicals
Alpha- and beta-carotene, caffeic acid, catechins, coumarin, cryptoxanthin, ferulic acid, isorhamnetin, limonene, lutein, phytoene, phytofluene, procyanidins, quercetin, ursolic acid, zeaxanthin

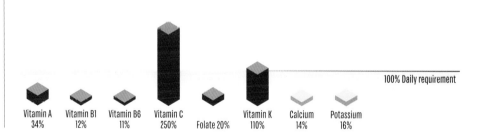

Vitamin A 34%	Vitamin B1 12%	Vitamin B6 11%	Vitamin C 250%	Folate 20%	Vitamin K 110%	Calcium 14%	Potassium 16%

100% Daily requirement

Star-Cressed Lovers

Bosc Berried Asparagus

Calories	207
Fat	1 g
Sat fat	0
Protein	4 g
Carbohydrate	53 g
Fiber	11 g

Asparagus is a powerful addition to any juice, and it has a mild flavor, which blends easily with other fruits and vegetables. As any asparagus lover can confirm, this vegetable possesses a natural diuretic compound. Many juicing chefs suggest that the entire stalk can be placed in the juicer, but the yield and taste are better if you break off the lower woody stem, as you do before cooking this vegetable. The Bosc pear is a hybrid variety with a slightly sweeter taste than the d'Anjou, and as it ripens, the taste becomes sweeter.

	1	cored medium Bosc pear (7 oz/200 g)
	4	medium spears asparagus (2 oz/60 g)
	½ cup (125 mL)	blackberries (2 oz/65 g)
	½ cup (125 mL)	red seedless grapes (2½ oz/75 g)

1. Wash all produce well. Using your hands, not a knife, break off lower stems of asparagus at the natural breaking point.

2. Place ingredients into juicer in order listed and juice.

Makes 1 serving (1 cup/250mL/240 g)

Phytochemicals
ALA, alpha- and beta-carotene, anthocyanidins, caffeic acid, catechins,chlorogenic acid, cyanidin, diosgenin, ellagic acid, friedelin, inositol, isorhamnetin, lignans, lutein, oleic acid, phenols, phytosterols, piceatannol, pterostilbene, resveratrol, stilbenoids, tannins, tartaric acid, ursolic acid

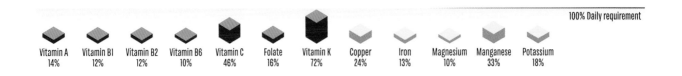

100% Daily requirement

Vitamin A	Vitamin B1	Vitamin B2	Vitamin B6	Vitamin C	Folate	Vitamin K	Copper	Iron	Magnesium	Manganese	Potassium
14%	12%	12%	10%	46%	16%	72%	24%	13%	10%	33%	18%

Cuked Carrot Berries

In juicing cucumbers, peeling isn't necessary, but doing so improves the taste by taking away some bitterness. You can also substitute pickling or Persian cucumbers, which don't have a bitter peel. The peel contains numerous phytochemicals, so it is advantageous to leave it on.

🍓	1 cup (250 mL)	hulled strawberries (4½ oz/130 g)
🥕	1	small carrot (2 oz/65 g)
🟤	¼	peeled medium pomegranate (2½ oz/70 g)
🥒	1	peeled small cucumber (5 oz/140 g)

1. Wash all produce well. Scrub carrot with a produce brush, but membranes of pomegranate are okay in the juicer.

2. Place ingredients into juicer in order listed and juice.

Makes 1 serving (1 cup/250 mL/245 g)

Calories	153
Fat	1 g
Sat fat	0
Protein	5 g
Carbohydrate	35 g
Fiber	8 g

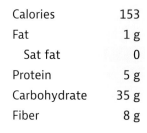

100% Daily requirement

Vitamin A 231%   Vitamin C 35%   Vitamin K 14%   No minerals present at 10% level.

Phytochemicals
ALA, alpha- and beta-carotene, bergapten, caffeic acid, campesterol, catechin, catechol, chlorogenic acid, coumarin, cryptoxanthin, cucurbitacin, cyanidin, ellagic acid, ferulic acid, gallic acid, geraniol, kaempferol, lupeol, lutein, luteolin, lycopene, matairesinol, pelargonidin, phytofluene, phytosterols,punicalagins, secoisolariciresinol, squalene, urosolic acid, zeaxanthin

Three-Berry Kumquat

Calories	225
Fat	2 g
Sat fat	0
Protein	7 g
Carbohydrate	51 g
Fiber	22 g

This recipe includes a trio of free-radical-fighting berries that create a sweet feast for the palate. While the berries contain some similar nutrients and phytochemicals, they also each possess an array of healthful compounds.

🍓	1 cup (250 mL)	hulled strawberries (5 oz/140 g)
🫐	1 cup (250 mL)	raspberries (4 oz/120 g)
🫐	¾ cup (175 mL)	blackberries (5 oz/140 g)
🍃	3	small kumquats (approx. 1½ oz/42 g each)
🥒	1	peeled medium cucumber (6½ oz/180 g)

1. Wash all produce well.

2. Place ingredients into juicer in order listed and juice.

Makes 1 serving (1 cup/250 mL/245 g)

Phytochemicals
ALA, alpha- and beta-carotene, bergapten, caffeic acid, campesterol, catechin, catechol, chlorogenic acid, coumarin, cryptoxanthin, cucurbitacin, cyanidin, ellagic acid, ferulic acid, gallic acid, geraniol, kaempferol, lupeol, lutein, luteolin, lycopene, matairesinol, pelargonidin, phytofluene, phytosterols, punicalagins, secoisolariciresinol, squalene, urosolic acid, zeaxanthin

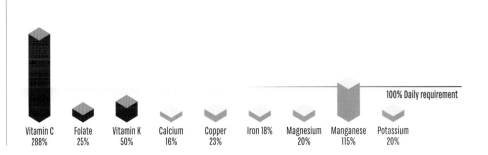

Vitamin C	Folate	Vitamin K	Calcium	Copper	Iron 18%	Magnesium	Manganese	Potassium
288%	25%	50%	16%	23%		20%	115%	20%

100% Daily requirement

Snipped Carrot Berries

The parsnip is a vegetable that, up until recently, didn't get much respect. That was before researchers started analyzing for phyto-chemicals. One such phytochemical, bergapten, possesses anticlotting and anti-inflammatory effects. In addition to parsnips, it is found in essential oils, especially from bergamot oranges and other citrus. Some juicer recipes don't call for peeling the parsnips, but the skin can be bitter.

	1 cup (250 mL)	raspberries (6 oz/120 g)
	3	large carrots (9½ oz/270 g)
	¼	medium parsnip (2½ oz/40 grams)

1. Wash all produce well. Scrub carrots and parsnip with a produce brush.

2. Place ingredients into juicer in order listed and juice.

Makes 1 serving (1 cup/250 mL/235 g)

Calories	214
Fat	1 g
Sat fat	0
Protein	5 g
Carbohydrate	49 g
Fiber	17 g

100% Daily requirement

Vitamin A	Vitamin C	Folate	Vitamin K	Calcium	Magnesium	Manganese	Potassium
935%	99%	13%	23%	11%	10%	52%	10%

Phytochemicals
ALA, alpha- and beta-carotene, anthocyanidins, bergapten, caffeic acid, campesterol, camphene, chlorogenic acid, coumarin, cryptoxanthin, ellagic acid, ferulic acid, geraniol, limonene, lupeol, luteolin, lycopene,myristicin, pelargonidin, phytofluene, phytosterols, quercetin, secoisolariciresinol

Red Pear Trio

Calories	214
Fat	1 g
Sat fat	0
Protein	4 g
Carbohydrate	54 g
Fiber	13 g

Raw beets work surprisingly well in juice recipes. In addition to the deep magenta color, it provides intriguing phytochemicals. One study in human subjects reported that the vegetable reduced inflammation and signs of oxidative damage. Beets are high in nitrate that the body converts to nitric oxide, which controls blood flow, muscle contraction and many other functions, so it may lower blood pressure and improve athletic performance.

Be sure to cut the top and bottom off the root, but save the greens for other recipes. The strawberry and pear blend well with the beet, and they add sweetness, as well as essential nutrients and more antioxidants and other phytochemicals.

🥬	½	beet (2 oz/52 g)
🍓	1½ cups (375 mL)	hulled strawberries (8 oz/225 g)
🍐	1	cored medium Bosc pear (7 oz/200 g)

1. Wash all produce well. Cut off top and bottom of beet; scrub with a produce brush.

2. Place ingredients into juicer in order listed and juice.

Makes 1 serving (1 cup/250 mL/240 g)

Phytochemicals
ALA, anthocyanidins, betaine, caffeic acid, catechin, catechol, chlorogenic acid, cyanidin, ellagic acid, friedelin, gallic acid, kaempferol, lutein, matairesinol, pelargonidin, phytosterols, secoisolariciresinol, tartaric acid, ursolic acid, zeaxanthin

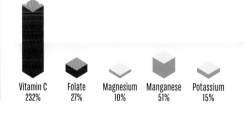

100% Daily requirement

Vitamin C	Folate	Magnesium	Manganese	Potassium
232%	27%	10%	51%	15%

Beeted Pear on the Vine

When studies first showed that people who consumed red wine had lower rates of heart disease, it wasn't clear what the beneficial compound might be. Since then, researchers have identified resveratrol as one of the keys. The good news for those who don't drink alcohol is that eating grapes, and especially drinking grape juice, offers the same advantage. Remember to use red or black grapes more often, though, as they contain the highest amounts of resveratrol.

1	beet (3½ oz/100 g)	
1¼ cups (300 mL)	black seedless grapes (7 oz/190 g)	
½	peeled large cucumber (4 oz/120 g)	
1	cored medium Bosc pear (7 oz/200 g)	

1. Wash all produce well. Cut off top and bottom of beet and scrub with a produce brush.

2. Place ingredients into juicer in order listed and juice.

Makes 1 serving (1⅓ cups/325 mL/325 g)

Calories	309
Fat	1 g
Sat fat	0
Protein	5 g
Carbohydrate	71 g
Fiber	12 g

Phytochemicals
ALA, anthocyanidins, betaine, caffeic acid, catechins, chlorogenic acid, cyanidin, cucurbitacin, ferulic acid, ellagic acid, friedelin, lutein, phytosterols, piceatannol, pterostilbene, resveratrol, squalene, tartaric acid, ursolic acid

100% Daily requirement

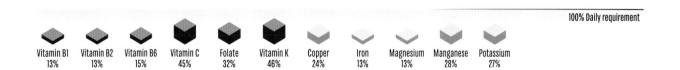

Vitamin B1	Vitamin B2	Vitamin B6	Vitamin C	Folate	Vitamin K	Copper	Iron	Magnesium	Manganese	Potassium
13%	13%	15%	45%	32%	46%	24%	13%	13%	28%	27%

Fruity Peppered Parsnips

Calories	268
Fat	1 g
Sat fat	0
Protein	3 g
Carbohydrate	68 g
Fiber	10 g

The sweet red bell pepper is the king of peppers for several reasons. While all peppers contain the important phytochemical capsaicin, from which their botanical name derives, the red bell pepper contains the highest level of carotenoid. One carotenoid in particular, lycopene, is important in prevention of prostate and breast cancer. This juice is a pleasant blend of the fruits and vegetables, although the sweetness of the fruits predominates.

	1 cup (250 mL)	seeded ribbed red bell pepper (3½ oz/100 g)
	¼	medium parsnip (2 oz/60 g)
	½ cup (125 mL)	red seedless grapes (2½ oz/75 g)
	1	cored large Bosc pear (8½ oz/240 g)

1. Wash all produce well. Scrub parsnip with a produce brush. pear.

2. Place ingredients into juicer in order listed and juice.

Makes 1 serving (1 cup/250 mL/295 g)

Phytochemicals
ALA, alpha-carotene, anthocyanidins, bergapten, caffeic acid, campesterol, camphene, capsaicin, catechins,chlorogenic acid, cinnamic acid, cryptoxanthin, cyanidin, ellagic acid, eugenol, friedelin, hesperidin, limonene, lutein, myristicin, phytoene, phytofluene, phytosterols, piceatannol, pterostilbene, quercetin, resveratrol, tartaric acid, ursolic acid, zeaxanthin

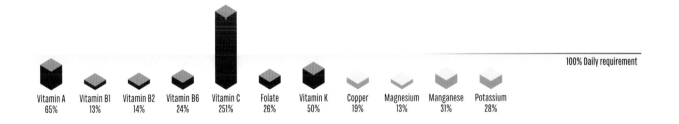

Vitamin A	Vitamin B1	Vitamin B2	Vitamin B6	Vitamin C	Folate	Vitamin K	Copper	Magnesium	Manganese	Potassium	100% Daily requirement
65%	13%	14%	24%	251%	26%	50%	19%	13%	31%	28%	

Pear Berry Pepper

This delicious juice contains an important phytochemical, ellagic acid. This compound's activities range from antioxidant, anti-inflammatory, antimicrobial and anticancer to protection against malaria and dental caries. Berries are one of the best sources for this important phytochemical. And raspberries make this juice fresh, sweet and tart.

Calories	208
Fat	2 g
Sat fat	0
Protein	4 g
Carbohydrate	51 g
Fiber	21 g

¼	seeded ribbed large green bell pepper (1½ oz/50 g)
½	cored large Bartlett pear (4 oz/120 g)
2 cups (500 mL)	raspberries (9 oz/250 g)

1. Wash all produce well.

2. Place ingredients into juicer in order listed and juice.

Makes 1 serving (¾ cup /175 mL/205 g)

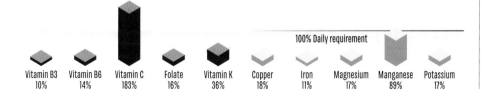

Vitamin B3	Vitamin B6	Vitamin C	Folate	Vitamin K	Copper	Iron	Magnesium	Manganese	Potassium
10%	14%	183%	16%	36%	18%	11%	17%	89%	17%

100% Daily requirement

Phytochemicals
ALA, alpha-carotene, anthocyanidins,caffeic acid, campesterol, capsaicin, chlorogenic acid, cinnamic acid, cryptoxanthin,cyanidin, ellagic acid, eugenol, friedelin, hesperidin, limonene, lutein, pelargonidin,phytoene, phytofluene, phytosterols, quercetin,ursolic acid, zeaxanthin

Kohlrabi Berry Kiwi

Calories	204
Fat	2 g
Sat fat	0
Protein	5 g
Carbohydrate	48 g
Fiber	11 g

Kohlrabi is a garden favorite, and as a member of the cruciferous family, it contains healthful phytochemicals. When juiced, it has a sharpish scent and a flavor that has a bit of a bite. You can use all parts of the plant, although this recipe only includes the bulb, which is not a true bulb but rather an extended stem. Not everyone on our tasting panel liked this juice, but most of us found it refreshing, especially when combined with this sweet trio of fruits.

	2	small kiwifruit (4 oz/115 g)
	½	medium kohlrabi (3½ oz/100 g)
	½ cup (125 mL)	blueberries (2½ oz/70 g)
	1	pitted medium nectarine (5 oz/140 g)

1. Wash all produce well. Cut off top and bottom of kohlrabi and scrub with a produce brush.

2. Place ingredients into juicer in order listed and juice.

Makes 1 serving (¾ cup/175 mL/200 g)

Phytochemicals
Alpha- and beta-carotene, anthocyanidin, caffeic acid, cathechin, chlorogenic acid, cryptoxanthin, cyanidin, ellagic acid, eugenol, ferulic acid, gallic acid, hydroxycinnamic acid, indoles, isothiocyanates, kaempferol, limonene, lutein, lycopene, myricetin, oleanolic acid, phytosterols, quercetin, rosmarinic acid, rutin, urosolic acid, zeaxanthin

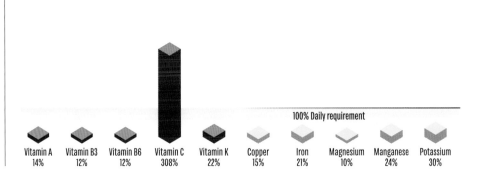

100% Daily requirement

Vitamin A	Vitamin B3	Vitamin B6	Vitamin C	Vitamin K	Copper	Iron	Magnesium	Manganese	Potassium
14%	12%	12%	308%	22%	15%	21%	10%	24%	30%

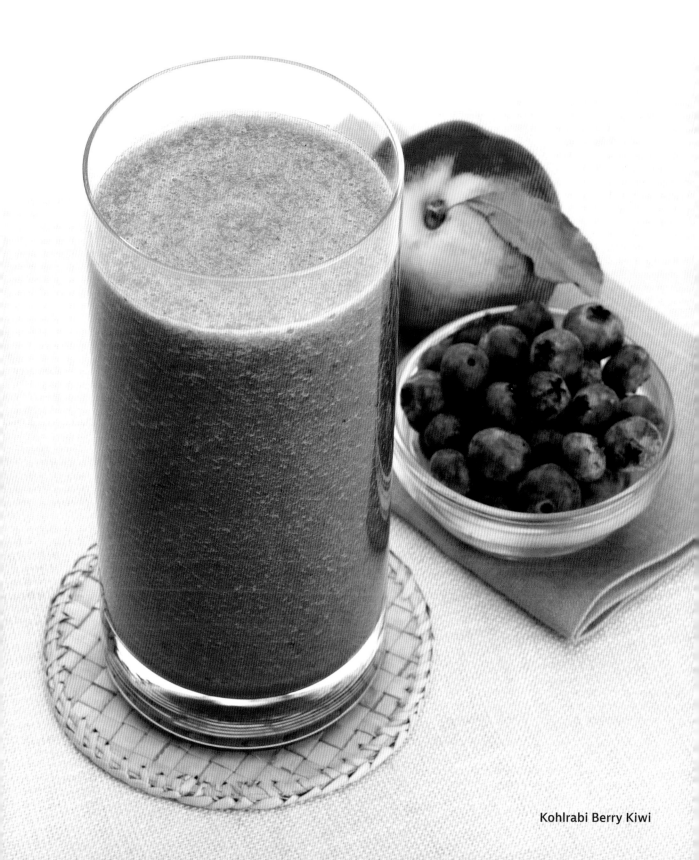

Kohlrabi Berry Kiwi

Green-Eyed Melon

Calories	163
Fat	1 g
Sat fat	0
Protein	3 g
Carbohydrate	40 g
Fiber	7 g

Super Enhancer Tip

The calories are low enough to add a tablespoon (15 mL) of either vanilla whey protein powder or fruit-flavored liquid protein to boost the protein content.

The horned melon is an intriguing-looking fruit, and we decided to try one in the juicer. One of its many names is blowfish, because of its resemblance to that creature. We tasted the peel to see if it was bitter, and it was not, so we didn't peel the fruit for this recipe. This makes it easier to use, since the spiny projections would make peeling difficult. It blends nicely with the fruits and beet greens in this recipe for a refreshing juice.

	1 cup (250 mL)	packed beet greens (1½ oz/40 g)
	½	medium horned melon (6 oz/160 g)
	½	cored large d'Anjou pear (4 oz/120 g)
	1	pitted medium peach (6 oz/150 g)

1. Wash all produce well.

2. Place ingredients into juicer in order listed and juice.

Makes 1 serving (1 cup/250 mL/210 g)

Phytochemicals

ALA, anthocyanidins, beta-sitosterol, caffeic acid, chlorogenic acid, cyanidin, ferulic acid, flavonols, friedelin, kaempferol, lutein, lycopene, oleic acid, quercetin, ursolic acid, zeaxanthin

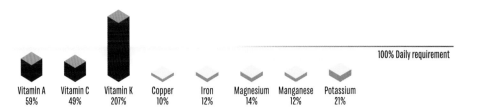

Vitamin A	Vitamin C	Vitamin K	Copper	Iron	Magnesium	Manganese	Potassium	100% Daily requirement
59%	49%	207%	10%	12%	14%	12%	21%	

Berry Green Citrus

This delicious blend of beet greens, berries and an orange is hard to beat in terms of taste and the nutrients and phytochemicals it provides. It makes a great start to any morning — and at only 185 calories, you can easily add some super enhancers to increase protein and add some fiber back in.

	1 cup (250 mL)	packed beet greens (1½ oz/40 g)
	1 cup (250 mL)	blackberries (4 oz/125 g)
	1	peeled medium orange (9 oz/260 g)

1. Wash all produce well.

2. Place ingredients into juicer in order listed and juice.

Makes 1 serving (¾ cup/175 mL/180 g)

Calories	185
Fat	1 g
Sat fat	0
Protein	5 g
Carbohydrate	44 g
Fiber	14 g

Super Enhancer Tips

Add 2 tbsp (30 mL) ground flaxseed to double the protein and put fiber — and omega-3 fats — back into the juice.

If you would prefer a sweeter taste with your protein and fiber, add 2 tbsp (30 ml) seed mixture instead of flax.

Phytochemicals

ALA, alpha- and beta-carotene, beta-sitosterol, caffeic acid, chlorogenic acid, coumarin, cryptoxanthin, cyanidin, ellagic acid, ferulic acid, isorhamnetin, kaempferol, lignans, limonene, lutein, oleic acid, phenolic acids, phytoene, phytofluene, quercetin, stilbenoids, tannins, zeaxanthin

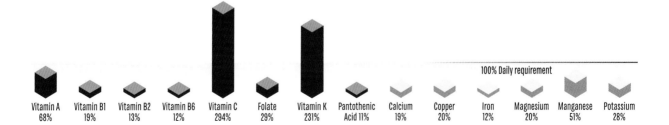

100% Daily requirement

Vitamin A	Vitamin B1	Vitamin B2	Vitamin B6	Vitamin C	Folate	Vitamin K	Pantothenic Acid	Calcium	Copper	Iron	Magnesium	Manganese	Potassium
68%	19%	13%	12%	294%	29%	231%	11%	19%	20%	12%	20%	51%	28%

Peppered Berry Juice

Calories	195
Fat	0
Sat fat	0
Protein	5 g
Carbohydrate	46 g
Fiber	10 g

Peppers are easy to grow in the summer garden, and a few plants can give an impressive yield. If you want to start a garden, this is one of the vegetables that is worth planting, since the cost can be quite high to buy them. The list of nutrients and phytochemicals make this delicious juice an excellent and quick start to the day.

🫑	½	seeded ribbed large green bell pepper (4 oz/110 g)
🍓	1 cup (250 mL)	hulled strawberries (5 oz/140 g)
🍊	1	peeled medium orange (9 oz/250 g)

1. Wash all produce well.

2. Place ingredients into juicer in order listed and juice.

Makes 1 serving (1 cup/250 mL/235 g)

Phytochemicals
ALA, alpha- and beta-carotene, caffeic acid, campesterol, capsaicin, catechins, catechol, chlorogenic acid, cinnamic acid, coumarin, cryptoxanthin, ellagic acid, eugenol, ferulic acid, gallic acid, hesperidin, kaempferol, limonene, lutein, matairesinol, pelargonidin, phytosterols, phytoene, phytofluene, quercetin, secoisolariciresinol, zeaxanthin

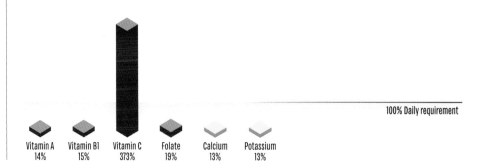

Vitamin A	Vitamin B1	Vitamin C	Folate	Calcium	Potassium
14%	15%	373%	19%	13%	13%

100% Daily requirement

Beet It, Tomato

The Honeycrisp apple is one of our favorites. It's a relative newcomer to the vast array of apple varieties, but the unique blend of sweetness and tartness make it a winner. Like most apples, it yields a high amount of juice.

1	cored large Honeycrisp apple (9 oz/260 g)
1 cup (250 mL)	red seedless grapes (6 oz/150 g)
1	medium beet (3½ oz/100 g)
1	large tomato (9 oz/260 g)

1. Wash all produce well. Cut off top and bottom of beet and scrub with a produce brush.

2. Place ingredients into juicer in order listed and juice.

Makes 2 servings (2 cups/500 mL/530 g)

Calories	165
Fat	0
Sat fat	0
Protein	3 g
Carbohydrate	41 g
Fiber	6 g

100% Daily requirement

Vitamin A	Vitamin C	Folate	Vitamin K	Manganese	Potassium
122%	56%	15%	18%	13%	22%

Phytochemicals
ALA, betaine, caffeic acid, campesterol, catechins, chlorogenic acid, chlorophyll, ellagic acid, eugenol, ferulic acid, isorhamnetin, lycopene, naringenin, phytoene, phytofluene, phytosterols, piceatannol, procyanidins, pterostilbene, quercetin, resveratrol, rutin, squalene, tartaric acid, ursolic acid, zeaxanthin

Mango Fandango

Calories	206
Fat	1 g
Sat fat	0
Protein	4 g
Carbohydrate	49 g
Fiber	6 g

The mango and orange blend extremely well, with both having some similar flavors but also complementing the other. The cucumber brings a light freshness to the juice, while the watercress adds an impressive array of nutrients and phytochemicals for few calories.

🥬	2 cups (500 mL)	packed watercress (3 oz/85 g)
🥒	½	peeled small cucumber (3 oz/85 g)
🥭	½	pitted medium mango (6 oz/175 g)
🍊	½	peeled medium orange (5 oz/140 g)

1. Wash all produce well. Remove excess stems from watercress.

2. Place ingredients into juicer in order listed and juice.

Makes 1 serving (1 cup/250 mL/250 g)

Phytochemicals
ALA, alpha- and beta-carotene, anacardic acid, caffeic acid, catechins, chlorogenic acid, coumarin, cryptoxanthin, cucurbitacin, ferulic acid, gallic acid, geraniol, kaempferol, limonene, lutein, mangiferin, phytoene, phytofluene, quercetin, squalene, tannins, zeaxanthin

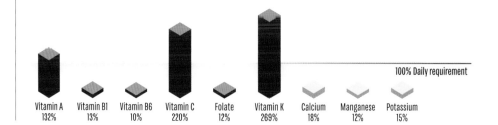

Vitamin A	Vitamin B1	Vitamin B6	Vitamin C	Folate	Vitamin K	Calcium	Manganese	Potassium
132%	13%	10%	220%	12%	269%	18%	12%	15%

100% Daily requirement

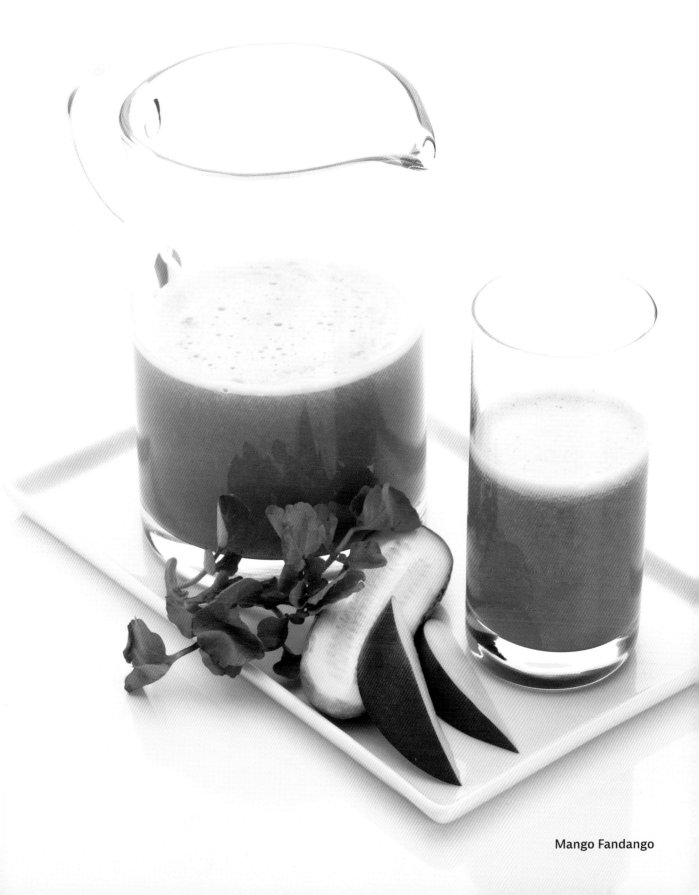

Mango Fandango

Blue Moon Zucchini

Calories	279
Fat	1 g
Sat fat	0
Protein	7 g
Carbohydrate	68 g
Fiber	11 g

This juice is higher in calories, so if you're trying to lose weight, you can dilute it with low-calorie almond milk or coconut water. But for everyone else, enjoy the tropical sweetness of this delicious drink.

🥒	2	small zucchini (7 oz/210 g)
🥕	1 cup (250 mL)	baby carrots (3½ oz/100 g)
🍍	1½ cups	peeled cored pineapple (8 oz/225 g)
🫐	1 cup (250 mL)	blueberries (5 oz/140 g)

1. Wash all produce well.

2. Place ingredients into juicer in order listed and juice.

Makes 1 serving (1 cup/250 mL/275 g)

Phytochemicals
Alpha- and beta-carotene, bergapten, caffeic acid, campesterol, cathechin, chlorogenic acid, coumarin, cryptoxanthin, cucurbitacin,cyanidin, ellagic acid, eugenol, ferulic acid, gallic acid, geraniol, isoflavones, limonene, lupeol, lutein, luteolin, lycopene, myricetin, oleanolic acid, phytofluene, phytosterols, quercetin, rosmarinic acid, rutin, secoisolariciresinol, urosolic acid, zeaxanthin

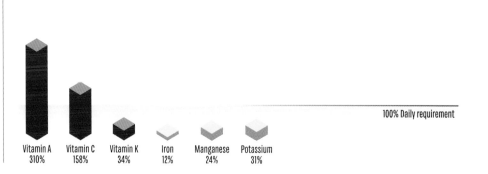

100% Daily requirement

Vitamin A	Vitamin C	Vitamin K	Iron	Manganese	Potassium
310%	158%	34%	12%	24%	31%

Beet Greens? Kwat the Heck?

Kumquats have been difficult to find in the past, but now they always seem to be available at large grocery stores. This is a boon for juicing, since these are the perfect fruit, needing only washing before extracting their nutrients and phytochemicals in the juicer. The flavors blend perfectly to produce a sweet juice with citrus undertones.

	Calories	208
	Fat	2 g
	Sat fat	0
	Protein	4 g
	Carbohydrate	51 g
	Fiber	21 g

	10	kumquats (approx. 3 oz/90 g each)
	2 cups (500 mL)	packed beet greens (3 oz/85 g)
	1	cored large Bartlett pear (9 oz/252 g)
	1 cup (250 mL)	hulled strawberries (5 oz/140 g)

1. Wash all produce well.

2. Place ingredients into juicer in order listed and juice.

Makes 1 serving (1¼ cups/300 mL/305 g)

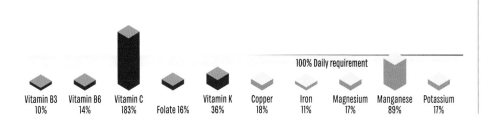

| Vitamin B3 10% | Vitamin B6 14% | Vitamin C 183% | Folate 16% | Vitamin K 36% | Copper 18% | Iron 11% | Magnesium 17% | Manganese 89% | Potassium 17% |

100% Daily requirement

Phytochemicals
ALA, anthocyanidins, beta-sitosterol, caffeic acid, catechins, catechol, chlorogenic acid, cyanidin, ellagic acid, ferulic acid, friedelin, gallic acid, hespertin, kaempferol, limonene, limonin, lutein, matairesinol, oleic acid, pelargonidin, phytoene, phytofluene, phytosterols, quercetin, secoisolariciresinol, ursolic acid, zeaxanthin

Snip It in the Bud

Calories	135
Fat	0
Sat fat	0
Protein	4 g
Carbohydrate	31 g
Fiber	8 g

Super Enhancer Tip

This recipe is lower in calories than many other juices, since it only contains vegetables. Try adding 2 tbsp (30 ml) of vanilla whey protein powder to boost protein, or if you prefer a less sweet-tasting juice, add 1 tbsp (15 ml) ground flaxseed.

Although this recipe includes only vegetables, the carrot provides enough sweetness to satisfy most palates. If you prefer a sweeter juice, adding a teaspoon (5 mL) of honey or other sweetener will do the trick. The lowly cucumber was considered by most people to be devoid of nutrients, but now scientists have shown that it contains many phytochemicals. One in particular, cucurbitacin, has anticancer effects. In addition, the cucumber is the perfect juicing ingredient when you need to increase the liquid. Try combining it with fruits or other vegetables that don't yield as much juice.

	⅓	large parsnip (3 oz/88 g)
	½	peeled small cucumber (3 oz/85 g)
	3	small carrots (4½ oz/126 g)

1. Wash all produce well. Scrub carrots and parsnip with a produce brush.

2. Place ingredients into juicer in order listed and juice.

Makes 1 serving (1 cup/250 mL/235 g)

Phytochemicals

ALA, alpha- and beta-carotene, bergapten, caffeic acid, campesterol, camphene, chlorogenic acid, coumarin, cryptoxanthin, cucurbitacin, ferulic acid, geraniol, limonene, lupeol, luteolin, lycopene, myristicin phytofluene, phytosterols, secoisolariciresinol, squalene

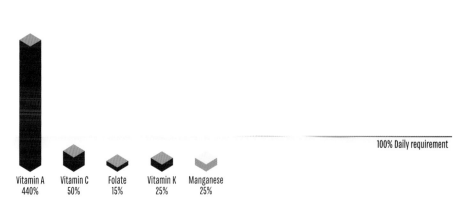

100% Daily requirement

Vitamin A 440% | Vitamin C 50% | Folate 15% | Vitamin K 25% | Manganese 25%

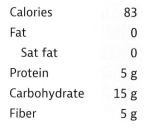

Pepperchini

The red bell pepper makes this recipe sweet enough without fruit, so it appeals to those who don't usually like vegetable juices. The nutritional benefits are numerous, starting with the low calories and the low carbohydrate content. The latter attribute makes it perfect for the person with prediabetes or diabetes, since it would count as 1 carbohydrate choice. For those who are trying to lose weight, a few tablespoons (about 2 tbsp/30 mL or ½ oz/16 g) of whey protein make the perfect meal swap.

Calories	83
Fat	0
Sat fat	0
Protein	5 g
Carbohydrate	15 g
Fiber	5 g

1 cup (250 mL)	seeded ribbed red bell pepper (3½ oz/100 g)	
1	peeled small cucumber (6 oz/170 g)	
1	baby zucchini (4 oz/110 g)	

1. Wash all produce well.

2. Place ingredients into juicer in order listed and juice.

Makes 1 serving (1 cup/250 mL/235 g)

Super Enhancer Tip

You can increase the protein by adding whey protein powder, seed mixture or ground flaxseed.

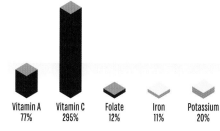

Vitamin A 77% Vitamin C 295% Folate 12% Iron 11% Potassium 20%

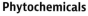

100% Daily requirement

Phytochemicals
ALA, alpha-carotene, caffeic acid, campesterol, capsaicin, chlorogenic acid, cinnamic acid, cryptoxanthin, cucurbitacin, eugenol, ferulic acid, hesperidin, isoflavones, limonene, lutein, phytoene, phytofluene, phytosterols, quercetin, secoisolariciresinol, squalene, zeaxanthin

Veggie Duo Delight

	JUICE	SOUP
Calories	101	161
Fat	1 g	1 g
Sat fat	0 g	0 g
Protein	7 g	10 g
Carb.	17 g	30 g
Fiber	3 g	6 g

Green pepper and tomato form the base for this delicious beverage, which can be enjoyed cold or hot. Make a double batch in the morning, drink half and use the other half for dinner soup. To make soup, coarsely process onions, carrots and basil and stir into juice, along with beans, and then heat.

Ingredients for Juicer

🫑	½	seeded ribbed large green bell pepper (4 oz/110 g)
🍅	1	medium tomato (7½ oz/210 g)
	2 tbsp (30 mL)	Greek yogurt (2 oz/55 g)

Additional Ingredients for Soup

🧅	⅓	medium sweet onion (2 oz/60 g)
🥕	¼ cup (60 mL)	baby carrots (1¼ oz/35 g)
🌿	¼ cup (60 mL)	fresh basil (¼ oz/6 g)
🫘	2 tbsp (30 ml)	black beans

1. Wash all produce well.

2. Place green pepper and tomato into juicer and juice.

3. Whisk in yogurt.

4. To make soup, coarsely chop vegetables and stir with black beans into juice.

Makes 1 serving juice (1 cup/250 mL/270 g) or 2 servings soup (2 cups/500 mL/540 g)

Phytochemicals (Juice)
ALA, alpha-carotene, caffeic acid, campesterol, capsaicin, chlorogenic acid, chlorophyll, cinnamic acid, cryptoxanthin, eugenol, ferulic acid, hesperidin, limonene, lutein, lycopene, naringenin, phytoene, phytofluene, phytosterols, quercetin, rutin, squalene, zeaxanthin

Additional Phytochemicals in Soup
anthocyanin, beta-carotene, bergapten, coumarin, geraniol, glucosinolates, isorhamnetin, kaempferol, lupeol, luteolin, oleanolic acid, secoisolariciresinol, saponin

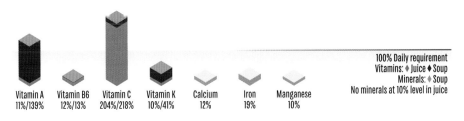

100% Daily requirement
Vitamins: ◆ Juice ◆ Soup
Minerals: ◆ Soup
No minerals at 10% level in juice

Vitamin A	Vitamin B6	Vitamin C	Vitamin K	Calcium	Iron	Manganese
11%/139%	12%/13%	204%/218%	10%/41%	12%	19%	10%

Soup's On Kohlrabi

The kohlrabi, tomato and carrot make for a dynamite vegetable juice for sipping. Make a double batch and save the other half for dinner. With the addition of some chopped vegetables and beans, it serves as a tasty soup base.

	JUICE	SOUP
Calories	122	185
Fat	0 g	1 g
Sat fat	0 g	0 g
Protein	5 g	8 g
Carb.	27 g	37 g
Fiber	8 g	11 g

Ingredients for Juicer

	½	medium kohlrabi (3½ oz/100 g)
	1	large tomato (9 oz/250 g)
	2	medium carrots (4 oz/113 g)

Additional Ingredients for Soup

	¼	medium onion (2 oz/55 g)
	¼ cup (60 mL)	fresh basil (¼ oz/6 g)
	¼ cup (60 ml)	chickpeas

1. Wash all produce well. Remove stems and leaves from kohlrabi; use a produce brush to clean carrots and kohlrabi.

2. Place vegetables into juicer in order listed and juice.

3. To make soup, coarsely chop vegetables and stir with chickpeas into juice

Makes 1 serving juice (1 cup/250 mL/270 g) or soup (1½ cups/375 mL/400 g)

Phytochemicals (Juice)
ALA, alpha- and beta-carotene, bergapten, caffeic acid, campesterol, chlorogenic acid, chlorophyll, coumarin, cryptoxanthin, eugenol, ferulic acid, geraniol, indoles, isothiocyanates, lupeol, luteolin, lycopene, naringenin, phytoene, phytofluene, phytosterols, quercetin, rutin, secoisolariciresinol, squalene, zeaxanthin

Additional Phytochemicals in Soup
Anthocyanin, caffeic acid, eugenol, gernaiol, glucosinolates, isorhamnetin, kaempferol, oleanolic acid, phytosterols, quercetin, rutin, saponin

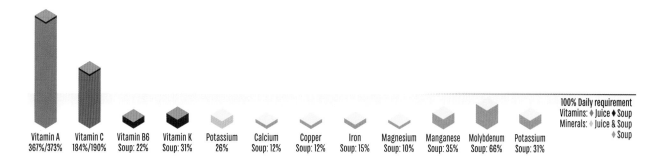

| Vitamin A 367%/373% | Vitamin C 184%/190% | Vitamin B6 Soup: 22% | Vitamin K Soup: 31% | Potassium 26% | Calcium Soup: 12% | Copper Soup: 12% | Iron Soup: 15% | Magnesium Soup: 10% | Manganese Soup: 35% | Molybdenum Soup: 66% | Potassium Soup: 31% |

100% Daily requirement
Vitamins: ♦ Juice ♦ Soup
Minerals: ♦ Juice & Soup
♦ Soup

Peaches 'n' Cream Oatmeal

Calories	176
Fat	2 g
Sat fat	0
Protein	8 g
Carbohydrate	33 g
Fiber*	5 g

*Fiber of pulp not included; this depends on pulp source)

This is the perfect type of recipe in which to include pulp, and if it was previously frozen, it will make this into a slushy. With protein, vitamins A and C and many phytochemicals, it makes a peachy breakfast when you're on the go.

1	pitted small peach (5 oz/140 g)
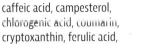 ½ cup	baby carrots (2½ oz/70 g)
1 tbsp (15 mL)	vanilla whey protein powder
1 tbsp (30 ml)	old-fashioned (large-flake) rolled oats
¼ cup (60 mL)	fruit pulp (see page 147)
½ cup (125 mL)	soy milk

1. Wash peach.

2. Add all ingredients to blender and process until desired consistency.

Makes 1 serving (1¼ cups/300 mL/340 g)

Phytochemicals
Alpha- and beta-carotene, anthocyanidin, bergapten, caffeic acid, campesterol, chlorogenic acid, coumarin, cryptoxanthin, ferulic acid, flavonols, geraniol, lupeol, lutein, luteolin, lycopene, phytofluene, phytosterols, quercetin, secoisolariciresinol, zeaxanthin

100% Daily requirement

Vitamin A 212%   Vitamin C 23%   Vitamin K 11%   No minerals present at 10% level

Peaches 'n' Cream
Oatmeal

Peppered Pasta

Calories	172
Fat	7 g
Sat fat	0
Protein	0
Carbohydrate	36 g
Fiber*	–

*Unable to determine
(pulp from peppers)

The pulp from some of the juiced vegetables makes an excellent base for many recipes (see opposite). You can save the pulp in the refrigerator for a day or so, but if you won't get to it before then, you should freeze it. We found that peppers yield the best pulp for any type of sautéed recipe, such as jazzing up vegetable or meat dishes. This recipe can be used as a base for pasta sauce by adding either fresh or canned tomatoes. It works well on its own to simply toss with some freshly boiled pasta. You can also mix it in with rice dishes.

	1 tbsp (15 mL)	olive oil
	½	large sweet onion (2½ oz/75 g)
	¼ cup (60 mL)	red bell pepper pulp (3 oz/80 g)
	¼ cup (60 mL)	green bell pepper pulp (3 oz/80 g)
	¼ cup (60 mL)	fresh basil (¼ oz/6 g)
		Whole-grain pasta or brown rice

1. Heat oil and sauté onion until softened.

2. Stir in the red and green pepper pulps until heated through, then stir in the fresh basil.

3. Toss with whole-grain pasta or brown rice.

Makes 2 servings (1 cup/250 mL/250 g sauce)

Phytochemicals
Anthocyanin, caffeic acid, eugenol, geraniol, glucosinolates, isorhamnetin, kaempferol, oleanolic acid, phytosterols, quercetin, rutin, saponin

All Things Pulp: Using Pulp in Recipes

Pulps from your juiced recipes can be saved and used in virtually any recipe. Make sure to label them, because you won't be able to remember what most of the pulps are just by looking at them. Refrigerate pulps promptly, and if you don't plan to use within a day or so, freeze them. You can sneak them into many of your favorite recipes with no adverse effects, and remember that you are using the healthful fiber that your juicer removed.

We found that the masticator-type juicer made a nicer pulp. It was more uniform and easier to incorporate into a wider variety of recipes. However, whichever type of juicer you use, remember to not waste this valuable source of fiber. Here are some suggestions for using pulp.

YOUR FAVORITE RECIPE	PULP AND AMOUNT	SUBSTITUTE FOR
Meatloaf (1½ to 2 lbs/ 675 g to 2 kg meat)	½ cup (125 mL) cup vegetable	Chopped vegetables
Stews (4 quarts/4 L)	1 cup (250 mL) vegetable	None needed
Soups (4 quarts/1 L)	1 cup (250 mL) vegetable	None needed
Pasta sauce (1 quart/1 L)	1 cup (250 mL) vegetable or fruit/ vegetable combo	None needed
Casseroles (9– by 11–inch/ 23 by 28 cm pan)	1 cup (250 mL) vegetable or fruit/ vegetable combo	None needed
Hot cereal (1 serving)	¼ cup (60 mL) fruit or vegetable	None needed
Blender smoothies	Any type and amount (pulp works well if frozen)	Up to half of fruit or vegetable
Quick breads and muffins (1 loaf pan or 12 muffins)	¼ cup (60 ml) fruit	Half of fruit or vegetable
Cakes and brownies	½ cup (125 mL) any type	None needed

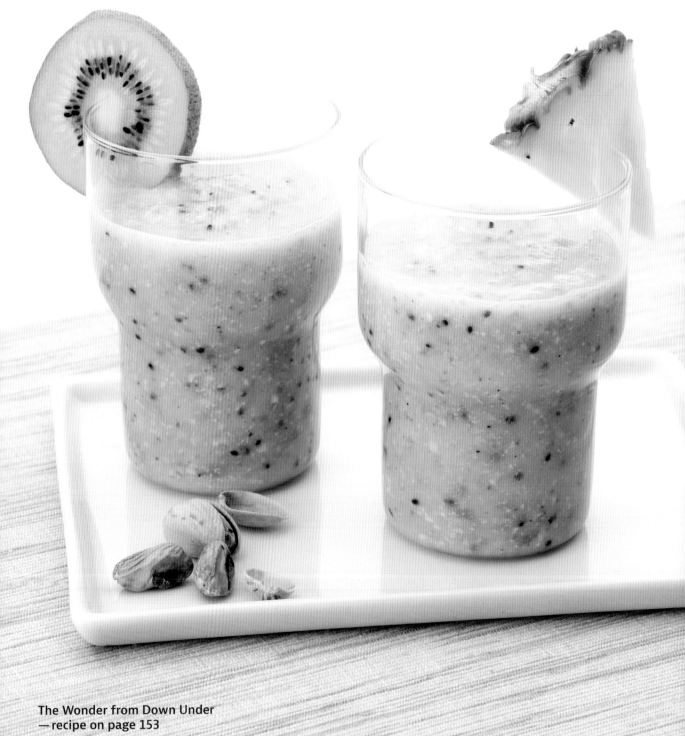

The Wonder from Down Under
— recipe on page 153

Blender/Food Processor Recipes

Sweet

Savory

The Wonder from Down Under

It's hard to beat the nutritional value of kiwi, and when you add pistachios and pineapple, the taste is also unbeatable. With the addition of nuts and almond milk, this makes a great breakfast on the run, since it provides protein and healthy fats to keep you feeling full all morning. The phytochemicals will fend off free radicals, and studies have shown that pistachios offer protection against cardiovascular disease in other ways, too.

Calories	296
Fat	14 g
Sat fat	0
Protein	7 g
Carbohydrate	41 g
Fiber	7 g

¼ cup (60 ml)	shelled unsalted pistachios (1¼ oz/34 g)
¼ cup (60 ml)	almond milk (⅓ oz/10 g)
2	peeled small kiwifruit (6½ oz/185 g)
½ cup (125 mL)	peeled cored fresh pineapple (5 oz/140 g)

1. In a blender, process nuts and almond milk.

2. Add pineapple and kiwi and blend.

Makes 1 serving (1½ cups/375 mL/300 g)

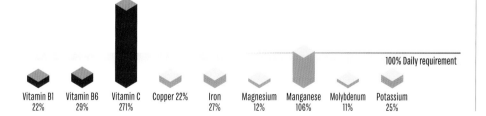

Vitamin B1	Vitamin B6	Vitamin C	Copper 22%	Iron	Magnesium	Manganese	Molybdenum	Potassium
22%	29%	271%		27%	12%	106%	11%	25%

100% Daily requirement

Phytochemicals
Cryptoxanthin, lutein, chlorogenic acid, ferulic acid, resveratrol, genistein, proanthocyanidins

Papakache Blend

Calories	166
Fat	0
Sat fat	0
Protein	2 g
Carbohydrate	43 g
Fiber	1 g

Super Enhancer Tip

One of our tasters preferred a slightly sweeter juice, although not everyone agreed. If you want to sweeten up the juice, add a product such as Super Seed Beyond Fiber, which contains stevia, a natural plant sweetener. Or if you have no objections, add either honey or sugar (or Splenda, which adds no calories).

Many people are not familiar with the wonderful texture and flavor of fresh papaya, and it's worth trying. Papaya is an incredibly nutrient-dense fruit, almost like a vegetable. Add to that the power of kale and tart cherries, and nutrition is off the charts. If you can't find baby kale, regular will serve very well. And tart cherries are hard to come by unless you live next to an orchard and can nab some during their short growing season, but this recipe uses frozen sour cherries, which are readily available. Many studies have been done on the benefits of tart cherries, which may even improve the condition of those with osteoarthritis.

	1 cup (250 mL)	peeled seeded papaya (5 oz/150 g)
	2 cups (500 mL)	packed baby kale (1 oz/30 g)
	1 cup (250 mL)	frozen sour cherries (5 oz/140 g)
	¼ cup (60 mL)	water

1. Wash all produce well.

2. Place all ingredients into blender and process until desired consistency.

Makes 2 servings (2 cups/500 mL/450 g)

Phytochemicals
Chlorogenic acid, cryptoxanthin, indole-3-carbinol, limonene, lutein, lycopene, proanthocyanidins, rutin, zeaxanthin

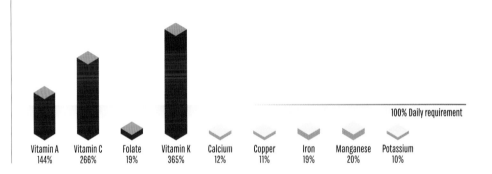

| Vitamin A 144% | Vitamin C 266% | Folate 19% | Vitamin K 365% | Calcium 12% | Copper 11% | Iron 19% | Manganese 20% | Potassium 10% |

100% Daily requirement

Bananaberry Soy Smoothie

This recipe combines the nutritional star power of three superfoods, and it's simple and delicious with only three main ingredients. Strawberries are high in vitamins A and C and loaded with fiber and antioxidants. The banana contributes vitamins C and B6, potassium, manganese and fiber, while soy adds protein, fiber and several antioxidants. Even though it is in an aseptic package (which means it does not require refrigeration until opened), silken tofu is usually found in the produce section of the grocery store.

	Calories	168
	Fat	2 g
	Sat fat	0
	Protein	7 g
	Carbohydrate	35 g
	Fiber	6 g

🍓	1 cup (250 mL)	hulled strawberries (5 oz/145 g)
	¼ cup (60 mL)	silken tofu (2 oz/60 g)
	1	peeled small banana (3½ oz/100 g)
	¼ cup (60 mL)	water

1. Cut strawberries in half and slightly mash banana.

2. Place all ingredients into blender and process until desired consistency.

Makes 1 serving (1½ cups/375 mL/365 g)

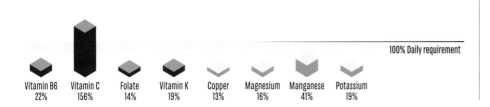

100% Daily requirement

Vitamin B6 22% Vitamin C 156% Folate 14% Vitamin K 19% Copper 13% Magnesium 16% Manganese 41% Potassium 19%

Phytochemicals
Kaempferol, pelargonidin, ellagic acid, gallic acid, chlorogenic acid, matairesinol, secoisolariciresinol, daidzein, genistein, glycitein, coumestrol, saponins, beta-sitosterol, inositol hexaphosphate, zeaxanthin

Orangey Creamsicle

Calories	98
Fat	1 g
Sat fat	0
Protein	7 g
Carbohydrate	18 g
Fiber	2 g

Super Enhancer Tips

👍 Add 1 tbsp (15 mL) vanilla whey protein powder for extra protein and more vanilla flavor.

👍 Since the calories are low, you can also add 1 tbsp (15 mL) ground flaxseed or seed mixture for a fiber boost.

This recipe is reminiscent of a frozen favorite from childhood. If you add a few ice cubes, it will be even more like that creamy orange treat on a stick.

1 cup (125 mL)	peeled seeded papaya (2½ oz/70 g)	
1 peeled	medium orange (7 oz/200 g)	
¼ cup (60 mL)	fat-free Greek yogurt (4 oz/115 g)	
¼ cup (60 mL)	soy milk	
½ tsp (2 mL)	pure vanilla extract	

Add all ingredients to blender and process until desired consistency.

Makes 2 servings (2 cups/500 mL/445 g)

Phytochemicals
ALA, alpha- and beta-carotene, coumarin, cryptoxanthin, ferulic acid, flavonols, limonene, lutein, lycopene, phytoene, phytofluene, tannins, zeaxanthin

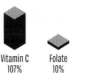

Vitamin C 107%	Folate 10%	Calcium 10%

100% Daily requirement

The Bee's Knees

Sweet potatoes bring vitamin A, iron and phytochemicals to this juice. When raw, they have a slightly bitter taste, though, so they work best when combined with a tart/sweet fruit, such as sour cherries. If you combine sweet potatoes with a sweeter fruit, you won't need to add a sweetener, which in this recipe is honey. Another alternative is to cook the sweet potatoes, which can be quickly done in a few minutes in the microwave. This will not affect the nutrients, since vitamin A, which is present in the highest amount, is not affected by heat.

Calories	168
Fat	3 g
Sat fat	0
Protein	4 g
Carbohydrate	34 g
Fiber	6 g

	½ cup (125 mL)	sweet potatoes (2 oz/60 g)
	1 cup (250 mL)	frozen sour cherries (4 oz/130 g)
	¼ cup (60 mL)	almond milk
	1 tbsp (15 mL)	ground flaxseed
	1 tsp (5 mL)	honey

1. Scrub sweet potato with a produce brush (leave skin on) and cut intro cubes.

2. Place ingredients into blender and process until desired consistency.

Makes 1 serving (1 cup/250 mL/250 g)

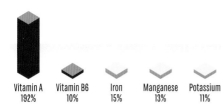

100% Daily requirement

Vitamin A 192% Vitamin B6 10% Iron 15% Manganese 13% Potassium 11%

Phytochemicals
ALA, beta-carotene, chlorogenic acid, matairesinol, neochlorogenic acid, limonene, lutein, phytoene, phytofluene, proanthocyanidins, rutin, secoisolariciresinol

Low-Cal Eye Opener

Calories	100
Fat	0
Sat fat	0
Protein	2 g
Carbohydrate	25 g
Fiber	3 g

Super Enhancer Tip

Since this juice is low in calories, add 2 tbsp (30 mL) vanilla whey protein powder for an even creamier smoothie that can replace a meal.

Papaya has a creamy quality, which makes a juice taste more substantial. It's also loaded with vitamins A and C and many phytochemicals. In this recipe, the cantaloupe, which is also high in these nutrients, adds liquid to provide volume and keep calories lower. But the real calorie saver is the broccoli, which brings nutrients and phytochemicals for very few calories.

	1 cup (250 mL)	peeled seeded papaya (3 oz/80 g)
	½ cup (125 mL)	broccoli florets (1¼ oz/37 g)
	1 cup (250 mL)	peeled seeded cantaloupe (5 oz/135 g)

1. Wash and trim broccoli, if required, to make small florets.

2. Place ingredients into blender and process until desired consistency.

Makes 1 serving (1 cup/250 mL/250 g)

Phytochemicals
ALA, alpha- and beta-carotene, caffeic acid, campesterol, chlorogenic acid, cryptoxanthin, ferulic acid, flavonols, indole-3-carbinol, isorhamnetin, kaempferol, lignan, lutein, lycopene, matairesinol, myricetin, phytoene, phytofluene, quercetin, sinigrin, sulforaphane, tannins, zeaxanthin

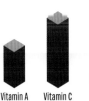

Vitamin A	Vitamin C	Folate	
126%	223%	22%	No minerals present at 10% level

100% Daily requirement

ABC Blend

This is a great juice for those trying to lose weight or people with diabetes. The calories are very low, and the carbohydrate count makes it 1 carbohydrate choice. The secret is arugula, a delicate-looking green that packs a wallop, both nutritionally and in taste. The flavor is often described as peppery, but it melds nicely with the two fruits in this juice. You can purchase baby arugula, which is the most tender and less bitter, in the produce section of most large grocery stores. Since it's considered a gourmet item, it can be a bit pricey. A better idea is to grow some for yourself, as it is one of the easiest superfoods to grow and takes minimal space in a garden. From planting to picking, it takes just 3 weeks, depending on the sunshine and rain.

Calories	74
Fat	1 g
Sat fat	0
Protein	3 g
Carbohydrate	16 g
Fiber	5 g

 1 cup (250 mL)   packed arugula (1 oz/28 g)

 ½ cup (125 mL)   peeled seeded cantaloupe (3 oz/80 g)

 ½ cup (125 mL)   blackberries (3 oz/85 g)

1. Wash all produce well. Cut cantaloupe into cubes.

2. Place ingredients into blender and process until desired consistency.

Makes 1 serving (¾ cup /175 mL/195 g)

100% Daily requirement

Vitamin A	Vitamin C	Folate	Vitamin K	Manganese
77%	85%	18%	58%	32%

Phytochemicals
ALA, alpha- and beta-carotene, caffeic acid, campesterol, cryptoxanthin, cyanidin,ellagic acid, ferulic acid, glucosinolates, indoles, isorhamnetin, lignans, lutein, phenolic acids, stilbenoids, sulforaphane,tannins, zeaxanthin

Tropical Breeze Smoothie

Calories	88
Fat	1 g
Sat fat	0
Protein	3 g
Carbohydrate	21 g
Fiber	4 g

Mango is a great fruit for juicing because it imparts creaminess and an intensely sweet flavor. Make sure the fruit is fully ripe before using it, as it will be fibrous and pungent if not ready for use. The mango is ripe when it gives slightly when pressed, and it will have a fruity aroma near the stem end. The sour cherries and broccoli add even more phytochemicals and lower the calorie level. You can use plain water to add liquid, but the coconut water adds additional antioxidants for few calories.

	½ cup (125 mL)	pitted mango (2½ oz/72 g)
	½ cup (125 mL)	broccoli florets (1½ oz/40 g)
	½ cup (125 mL)	frozen sour cherries (2¼ oz/63 g)
	¼ cup (60 mL)	coconut water

1. Wash all produce well. Leave skin on mango and cut into chunks.

2. Place ingredients into blender and process until desired consistency.

Makes 1 serving (1 cup/250 mL/235 g)

Phytochemicals
Alpha- and beta-carotene, anacardic acid, caffeic acid, catechins, chlorogenic acid, cryptoxanthin, ferulic acid, gallic acid, geraniol, indole-3 carbinol, isorhamnetin, kaempferol, lignan, limonene, lutein, mangiferin, matairesinol, myricetin, naringenin, proanthocyanidins, quercetin, rutin, sinigrin, sulforaphane, tannins

  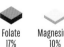 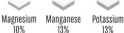

100% Daily requirement

Vitamin A	Vitamin B6	Vitamin C	Folate	Magnesium	Manganese	Potassium
49%	10%	109%	17%	10%	13%	13%

Apple Berry Pepper

This juice comes in below 100 calories per serving, so it will work well for a calorie-cutting regimen, and it is diabetes-friendly, providing about 1 carbohydrate exchange. Although it's light on calories and carbs, it's not light on taste, with a sweet blend of nutrient-dense fruits and vegetables.

Calories		77
Fat		1 g
Sat fat		0
Protein		1 g
Carbohydrate		17 g
Fiber		5 g

	½ cup (125 mL)	seeded ribbed red bell pepper (1½ oz/45 g)
	¼	cored medium Fuji apple (2 oz/60 g)
	¼ cup (60 mL)	blackberries (1¼ oz/35 g)
	¼ cup (60 mL)	almond milk
	¼ tsp (1 mL)	ground cinnamon

1. Wash all produce well and cut into chunks.

2. Place ingredients into blender and process.

Makes 1 serving (¾ cup /175 mL/205 g)

Super Enhancer Tips

Whisk in an additional ¼ tsp (1 mL) cinnamon for additional phytochemicals and a great flavor. Blackberries stand up quite well to this aromatic spice.

Add 1 tbsp (15 mL) ground flaxseed and ½ tbsp (7 mL) seed mixture; you'll have even more protein and nutrients without too many extra calories.

Phytochemicals

AI A. alpha-carotene. caffeic acid, campesterol, capsaicin, catechins, chlorogenic acid, cinnamic acid, coumarin ,cyanidin,cryptoxanthin, ellagic acid, eugenol, ferulic acid, geraniol, hesperidin, isorhamnetin,lignans, limonene, lutein, phenolic acids, phytoene, phytofluene, phytosterols, procyanidins, quercetin, stilbenoids, tannins, ursolic acid, zeaxanthin

100% Daily requirement

Vitamin A 35% Vitamin C 117% Vitamin K 12% Manganese 14%

Broccoberry Smoothie

Calories	100
Fat	1 g
Sat fat	0
Protein	3 g
Carbohydrate	20 g
Fiber	5 g

Super Enhancer Tip

Add ¾ tbsp (12 mL) unsweetened cocoa powder; dark cocoa is best for maximum antioxidants.

Strawberries blend nicely with papaya, and both will make you forget you're getting a serving of broccoli! Remember that you can easily substitute any type of milk for the soy milk, including low-fat or skim milk. The touch of milk will go well with the Super Enhancer Tip of whisking in some dark cocoa. While most people prefer to drink cold juices and smoothies, heating this one up makes it a great morning beverage.

½ cup (125 mL)	hulled strawberries (2½ oz/75 g)
½ cup (125 mL)	peeled seeded papaya (2¼ oz/70 g)
½ cup (125 mL)	broccoli florets (1¼ oz/36 g)
2 tbsp (30 mL)	soy milk

1. Wash all produce well.

2. Place all ingredients in blender and process until desired consistency.

Makes 1 serving (¾ cup/175 mL/210 g)

Phytochemicals

ALA, caffeic acid, catechins, catechol, chlorogenic acid, cryptoxanthin, ellagic acid, ferulic acid, gallic acid, flavonols, indole-3-carbinol, isorhamnetin, kaempferol, lignan, lutein, lycopene, matairesinol, myricetin, pelargonidin, phytoene, phytofluene, phytosterols, quercetin, sinigrin, sulforaphane, secoisolariciresinol, tannins, zeaxanthin

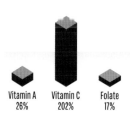

100% Daily requirement

Vitamin A 26%   Vitamin C 202%   Folate 17%   Manganese 22%

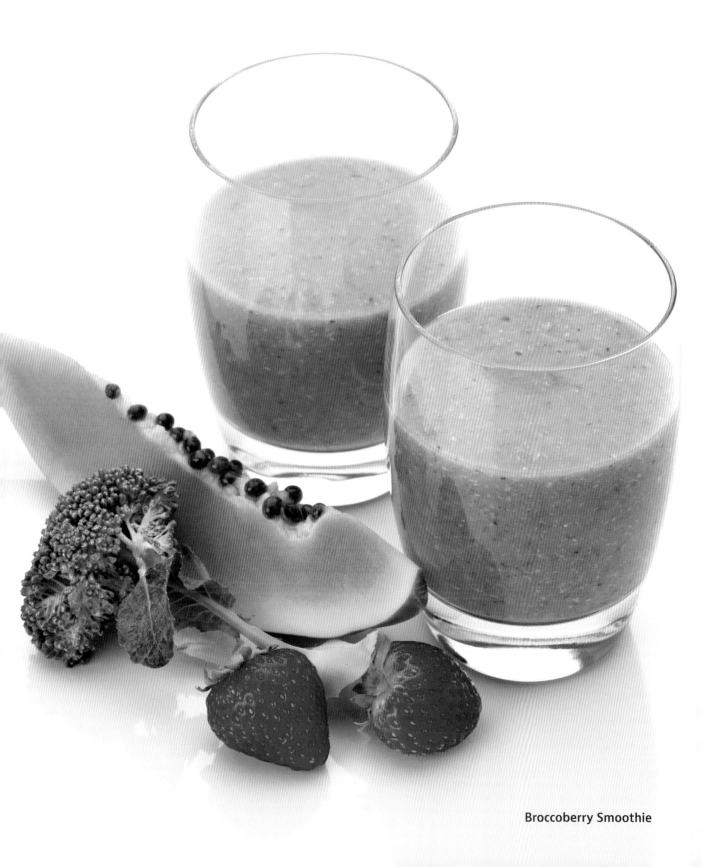

Broccoberry Smoothie

Citrus Bapple

Calories	85
Fat	1 g
Sat fat	0
Protein	1 g
Carbohydrate	21 g
Fiber	4 g

Super Enhancer Tip

👍 Add ½ tbsp (7 mL) seed mix to add fiber and protein and a touch of extra sweetness.

You can use any type of grapefruit in these recipes, but we prefer the red or pink for the higher carotenoid content, specifically lycopene. Since the carrots and strawberries also add this extraordinary antioxidant, the juice is a superb source of this vital phytochemical. While most people are aware of lycopene's protection against prostate cancer, studies have more recently pointed to its anti-inflammatory effects.

🍊	½ cup (125 mL)	peeled seeded red or pink grapefruit segments (2½ oz/70 g)
🥕	¼ cup (60 mL)	baby carrots (1¼ oz/35 g)
🍓	½ cup (125 mL)	hulled strawberries (3 oz/77 g)
🍎	¼ cup (60 mL)	cored Red Delicious apple (1¼ oz/33 g)

1. Wash all produce well and cut into chunks.

2. Add to blender and process to desired consistency, adding water if too thick.

Makes 1 serving (¾ cup /175 mL/220 g)

Phytochemicals

ALA, alpha- and beta-carotene, bergapten, caffeic acid, campesterol, catechins, catechol, chlorogenic acid, coumarin, cryptoxanthin, ellagic acid, ferulic acid, gallic acid, geraniol, hesperetin, hesperidin, isorhamnetin, kaempferol, limonene, lupeol, lutein, luteolin, lycopene, matairesinol, pelargonidin, phytofluene, phytosterols, procyanidins, quercetin, secoisolariciresinol, ursolic acid, zeaxanthin

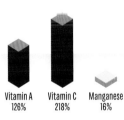

100% Daily requirement

Vitamin A 126% Vitamin C 218% Manganese 16%

Mango Tango

This recipe is a perfect combination of fruits and vegetables to yield both taste and a great nutritional and phytochemical profile. The mango, orange and arugula contribute vitamins A and C, while important phytochemicals come from the cucumber and apple.

	½ cup (125 mL)	pitted mango (2½ oz/78 g)
	½ cup (125 mL)	cored apple (2¼ oz/65 g)
	½ cup (125 mL)	peeled cucumber (2 oz/56 g)
	1 cup (250 mL)	packed arugula (1 oz/28 g)
	2 tbsp (30 mL)	coconut water

1. Wash all produce well. Peel only the cucumber.

2. Place all ingredients in blender and process until desired consistency.

Makes 1 serving (1 cup/250 mL/260 g)

Calories	102
Fat	1 g
Sat fat	0
Protein	2 g
Carbohydrate	25 g
Fiber	4 g

Super Enhancer Tip

Add 1 tbsp (15 mL) vanilla whey protein powder to increase protein and enhance the taste.

100% Daily requirement

Vitamin A	Vitamin C	Folate	Vitamin K	Manganese	Potassium
34%	67%	15%	35%	10%	11%

Phytochemicals
ALA, alpha- and beta-carotene, anacardic acid, caffeic acid, catechins, chlorogenic acid, cucurbitacin, cryptoxanthin, ferulic acid, gallic acid, glucosinolates, indoles, isorhamnetin, kaempferol, lutein, mangiferin, procyanidins, quercetin, squalene, sulforaphane, tannins, ursolic acid, zeaxanthin

Cantaloupe Island

Calories	178
Fat	9 g
Sat fat	0
Protein	4 g
Carbohydrate	24 g
Fiber	5 g

The cantaloupe is one of those fruits with the nutritional profile of a vegetable. It's perfect for juicing because it provides lots of liquid and sweetness. To maximize the sweetness, make sure to leave the cantaloupe on the counter to ripen before using it. Turn it every now and again so that no mold spots develop as it ripens. You'll notice a fragrant aroma, especially at the stem end, when it is ready.

	¾ cup (175 mL)	peeled seeded cantaloupe (3½ oz/105 g)
	⅓ cup (75 mL)	peeled banana (1 oz/28 g)
	½ cup (125 mL)	peeled cucumber (2 oz/56 g)
	½ cup (125 mL)	blackberries (2½ oz/74 g)
	2 tbsp (30 ml)	walnuts (½ oz/13 g)

1. Wash all produce well.

2. Place all ingredients in blender and process until desired consistency.

Makes 1 serving (1¼ cups/300 mL/300 g)

Phytochemicals
ALA, alpha- and beta-carotene, caffeic acid, campesterol, chlorogenic acid, cryptoxanthin, cucurbitacin, cyanidin, ellagic acid, ferulic acid, inositol, isorhamnetin, lignans, lutein, kaempferol, pelargonidin, phenolic acids, phytosterols, quercetin, rutin, squalene, stilbenoids, tannins

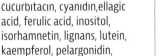
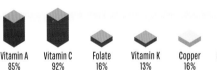

100% Daily requirement

Vitamin A	Vitamin C	Folate	Vitamin K	Copper	Manganese
85%	92%	16%	13%	16%	42%

Tofu Tart

This recipe is a low-calorie and low-carbohydrate treat. Although the essential nutrients appear to be low (with the exception of vitamin A), you'll notice that the phytochemicals are abundant. This is especially true for two of the ingredients, tofu and tart cherries. The tofu provides the important isoflavone and phytosterol compounds. Studies show that these compounds provide protection against cancer and cardiovascular disease. And the sour cherries are almost considered a medicine for the antioxidant and anti-inflammatory power wrapped up in this tiny fruit.

	½ cup (125 mL)	frozen sour cherries (2½ oz/70 g)
	¼ cup (60 ml)	baby carrots (1¼ oz/35 g)
	¼ cup (60 ml)	extra-firm silken tofu (1½ oz/42 g)
	2 tbsp (30 mL)	coconut water (1 fl oz/30 mL)
	½ tsp (1 mL)	honey

Place all ingredients in blender and process until desired consistency.

Makes 1 serving (¾ cup/175 mL/180 g)

Calories	71
Fat	1 g
Sat fat	0
Protein	4 g
Carbohydrate	12 g
Fiber	2 g

Super Enhancer Tip

To add more essential nutrients, consider adding a tablespoon (15 mL) of seed mixture.

Vitamin A
132%   No minerals present at 10% level

100% Daily requirement

Phytochemicals
Alpha- and beta-carotene, bergapten, caffeic acid, campesterol, chlorogenic acid, coumarin, cryptoxanthin, ferulic acid, geraniol, isoflavones, lignan, limonene, lupeol, luteolin, lycopene, naringenin, phytofluene, phytosterols, proanthocyanidins, rutin, secoisolariciresinol

Choco Chickie

Calories	151
Fat	2 g
Sat fat	0
Protein	5 g
Carbohydrate	30 g
Fiber	3 g

Super Enhancer Tip

Add 2 tbsp (30 mL), or ½ oz (13 g), walnuts for protein, fiber and important phytochemicals.

The banana is a wonderful juicing fruit, but you will need other ingredients with more liquid, and the same is true for chickpeas. In this recipe, cantaloupe provides the liquid, along with vitamins A and C. If you enjoy the taste of cocoa powder, you can increase the amount, although it can add bitterness at higher levels. The calories and protein are at a perfect level to make this a take-along breakfast treat.

	¼ cup (60 mL)	chickpeas (1½ oz/40 g)
	¼ cup (60 ml)	banana chunks (1¾ oz/47 g)
	¼ cup (60 mL)	peeled seeded cantaloupe (2½ oz/74 g)
	2 tbsp (30 mL)	almond milk
	1 tbsp (15 mL)	unsweetened cocoa powder

Place all ingredients in blender and process until desired consistency.

Makes 1 serving (¾ cup/175 mL/190 g)

Phytochemicals
ALA, alpha- and beta-carotene, caffeic acid, campesterol, catechins, coumarin, cryptoxanthin, cucurbitacin, cyanidins, ferulic acid, flavonols, gallic acid, inositol, kaempferol, lutein, methylxanthines,pelargonidin, phytosterols, proanthocyanidins, quercetin, rutin, tannins, theaflavins, trigonelline

100% Daily requirement

Vitamin A 57%   Vitamin C 51%   Folate 12%   Manganese 22%

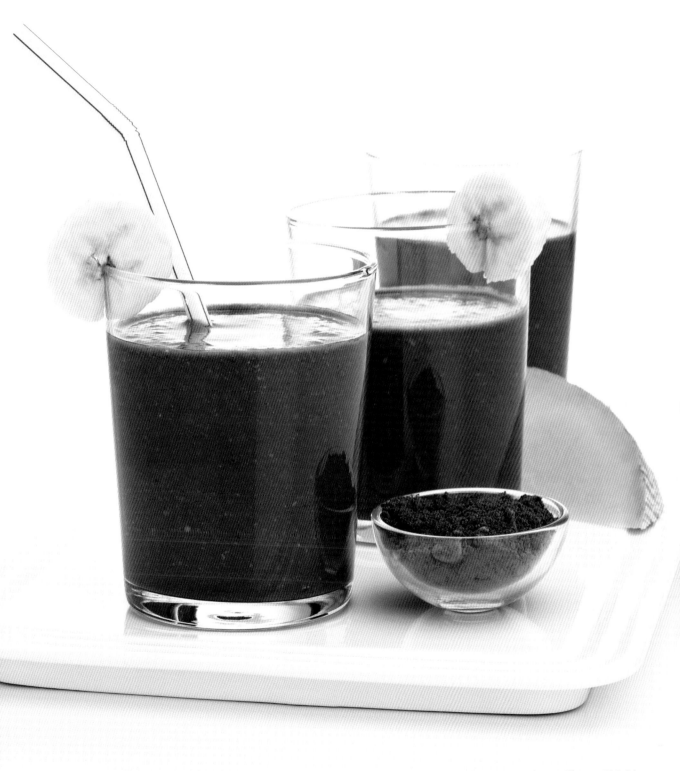

Choco Chickie

Apple Pie

Calories	90
Fat	3 g
Sat fat	0
Protein	6 g
Carbohydrate	12 g
Fiber	2 g

Super Enhancer Tips

Add a tablespoon or two (15 to 30 mL) of vanilla whey protein powder.

Add a tablespoon (15 mL) of ground flaxseed or seed mixture for a protein and fiber boost.

If you love cinnamon, you can increase the amount for additional phytochemicals.

This is another recipe that at first glance appears to be low in nutrients. However, it contains key phytochemicals that you won't get from other sources. In addition, it provides good-quality protein, and you can boost that by adding vanilla whey protein.

This recipe includes tofu, and we prefer the silken variety, particularly the type that is aseptically packaged. The packaging makes it shelf stable and it only requires refrigeration after opening.

½ cup (125 mL)	cored Fuji apple (2½ oz/76 g)
¼ cup (60 mL)	extra-firm silken tofu (1½ oz/42 g)
2 tbsp (30 mL)	almond milk
2 tbsp (30 mL)	water
½ tsp (2 mL)	honey
¼ tsp (1 mL)	apple pie spice (or cinnamon, nutmeg and allspice)

1. Wash apple but leave skin on.

2. Place all ingredients in blender and process until desired consistency.

Makes 1 serving (¾ cup/175 mL/195 g)

Phytochemicals
Catechins, caffeic acid, ferulic acid, isoflavones, isorhamnetin, lignans, phytosterols, procyanidins, quercetin, ursolic acid

No vitamins present at 10% level

Calcium 10% · Manganese 45% · Potassium 13%

100% Daily requirement

Pumpkin Pie

This is a fun recipe with many nutritional benefits. It contains plenty of protein to serve as a meal, although it tastes like dessert. Don't be put off by the high fat content, because it's in the form of healthy fats — unsaturated. The vitamin A level, at over five times what you need in a day, is in the form of beta-carotene, the antioxidant extraordinaire.

	½ cup (125 mL)	baby carrots (2 oz/58 g)
	⅓ cup (75 mL)	extra-firm silken tofu (2 oz/60 g)
	4 tbsp (60 mL)	almond milk
	6 tbsp (90 mL)	water
	½ cup (125 mL)	canned 100% pumpkin purée (4½ oz/128 g)
	2 tbsp (30 mL)	walnuts (½ oz/16 g)
	1 tsp (5 mL)	honey
	½ tsp (2 mL)	ground cinnamon

1. Place carrots, tofu, almond milk and water in blender and process.

2. Add pumpkin, walnuts, honey and cinnamon; pulse (use the stop/start toggle switch) several times, until desired consistency.

Makes 2 servings (1¾ cups/400 mL/405 g)

Calories	229
Fat	14 g
Sat fat	0
Protein	11 g
Carbohydrate	20 g
Fiber	6 g

Super Enhancer Tip

Okay, we admit that this doesn't do much for the nutrient profile, but you should try this with a dash of whipped cream!

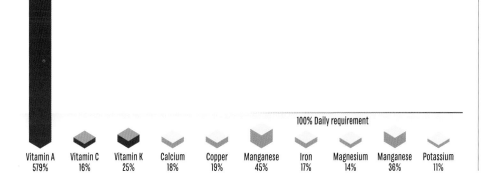

| Vitamin A 579% | Vitamin C 16% | Vitamin K 25% | Calcium 18% | Copper 19% | Manganese 45% | Iron 17% | Magnesium 14% | Manganese 36% | Potassium 11% |

100% Daily requirement

Phytochemicals
ALA, alpha- and beta-carotene, bergapten, caffeic acid, campesterol, chlorogenic acid, coumarin, cryptoxanthin, ferulic acid, geraniol, lignans, lupeol, luteolin, lycopene, phytofluene, phytosterols, secoisolariciresinol

Bananaloupe Veggie

Calories	131
Fat	1 g
Sat fat	0
Protein	3 g
Carbohydrate	33 g
Fiber	5 g

Super Enhancer Tip

Add 2 tsp (10 mL) chia seeds for more ALA, fiber and protein.

These ingredients may seem an unlikely combination, but both the tomato and broccoli lend themselves quite well to being blended with the sweet fruits. The nutritional scorecard is fantastic, with the banana providing vitamin B6 and the orange fruits providing both vitamin A and C. In addition, this recipe boasts an incredible list of phytochemicals.

	½	peeled medium banana (2 oz/58 g)
	¼ cup (60 mL)	peeled seeded cantaloupe (1½ oz/40 g)
	½ cup (125 mL)	broccoli florets (1¾ oz/47 g)
	½ cup (125 mL)	peeled seeded papaya (3 oz/80 g)
	½	medium tomato (2 oz/55 g)

Add all ingredients to blender and process until desired consistency.

Makes 1 serving (1 cup/250 mL/280 g)

Phytochemicals

ALA, alpha- and beta-carotene, caffeic acid, campesterol, chlorogenic acid, chlorophyll, cryptoxanthin, cucurbitacin, cyanidins, eugenol, ferulic acid, flavonols, indole-3-carbinol, inositol, isorhamnetin, kaempferol, lignan, lutein, lycopene, matairesinol, myricetin, naringenin, pelargonidin, phytoene, phytofluene, phytosterols, quercetin, rutin, sinigrin, sulforaphane, squalene, tannins, zeaxanthin

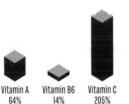

100% Daily requirement

Vitamin A	Vitamin B6	Vitamin C	Folate	Manganese	Potassium
64%	14%	205%	20%	13%	10%

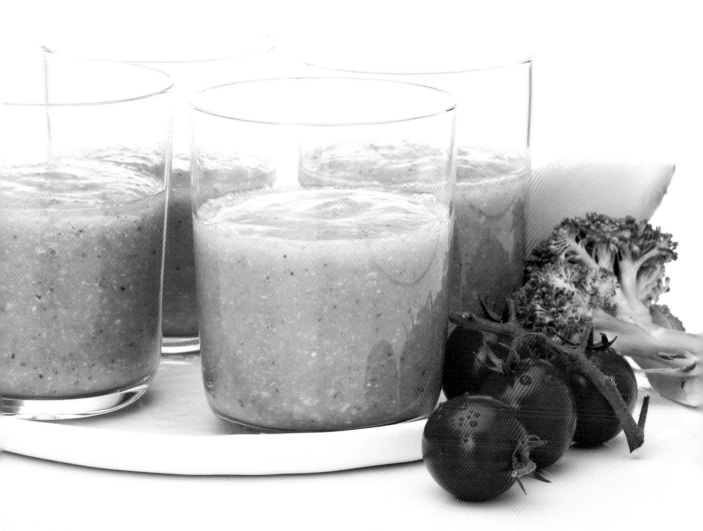

Bananaloupe Veggie

Blueberry Muffin

Calories	178
Fat	4 g
Sat fat	0
Protein	7 g
Carbohydrate	35 g
Fiber	8 g

It's hard to beat the health effects of blueberries, with numerous studies focusing specifically on this berry. This recipe adds the power of the berries to the phytochemicals from tofu. We added some kefir labne, though Greek yogurt will work just as well, and this adds some probiotics to the mix. But the best part of this recipe is the taste. In fact, after drinking it for a nice lunch, we served some later in the day with a dollop of whipped cream as a dessert. As with most blended smoothies, this one thickens after being refrigerated.

	½	peeled medium banana (2 oz/54 g)
	1 cup (250 mL)	blueberries (5 oz/150 g)
	⅓ cup (75 mL)	extra-firm silken tofu (2 oz/60 g)
	2 tbsp (30 mL)	kefir cheese (labne) or nonfat Greek yogurt
	¼ cup (60 mL)	soy milk
	1 tsp (5 mL)	pure vanilla extract

Place all ingredients in blender and process until desired consistency.

Makes 1 serving (1½ cups/375 mL/355 g)

Phytochemicals
ALA, alpha- and beta-carotene, caffeic acid, cathechin, chlorogenic acid, cryptoxanthin, campesterol, cyanidin,ellagic acid, eugenol, ferulic acid, gallic acid, hydroxycinnamic acid, inositol, kaempferol, lutein, limonene, myricetin, oleanolic acid, pelargonidin, phytosterols, quercetin, rosmarinic acid, rutin, urosolic acid

100% Daily requirement

Vitamin B6	Vitamin C	Calcium	Iron	Magnesium	Potassium
10%	60%	11%	10%	10%	11%

Double Berry Dew

In addition to adding sweetness, dates bring important nutrients and phytochemicals to the recipe. The two varieties that are most available are Medjool, which are large and rounded, and the date palm, smaller and more slender. One study on dates showed that they lowered the level of triglyceride (fat) in the blood and provided important protection against heart disease. Since this recipe is a bit higher in calories, you may opt to consider it as 2 servings. You can drink half in the morning and save the other half for a fragrant dessert with dinner.

Calories	197
Fat	1 g
Sat fat	0
Protein	3 g
Carbohydrate	52 g
Fiber	7 g

	⅓ cup (75 mL)	peeled seeded papaya (2½ oz/74 g)
	¼ cup (60 mL)	blackberries (1½ oz/40 g)
	¼ cup (60 mL)	hulled strawberries (1¼ oz/34 g)
	1 cup (500 mL)	peeled seeded honeydew melon (5 oz/140 g)
	3	dates (1 oz/28 g each)
	¼ cup (60 mL)	coconut water

1. Wash all produce well and cut into chunks.

2. Place all ingredients in blender and process until desire consistency.

Makes 1 serving (1½ cups /375 mL/375 g)

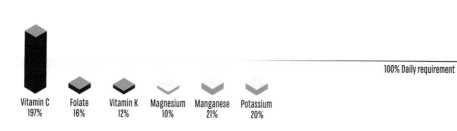

Vitamin C 197%   Folate 16%   Vitamin K 12%   Magnesium 10%   Manganese 21%   Potassium 20%

100% Daily requirement

Phytochemicals
ALA, alpha- and beta-carotene, caffeic acid, campesterol, catechins, catechol, chlorogenic acid, cryptoxanthin, cucurbitacin, cyanidin, ellagic acid, ferulic acid, flavonols, gallic acid, isorhamnetin, kaempferol, lignans, lutein, lycopene, matairesinol, pelargonidin, phenolic acids, phytoene, phytofluene, phytosterols, secoisolariciresinol, stilbenoids, tannins, zeaxanthin

Tutti Fruitti

Calories	99
Fat	1 g
Sat fat	0
Protein	2 g
Carbohydrate	23 g
Fiber	4 g

Super Enhancer Tips

Try this with either fruit-flavored liquid protein or vanilla whey protein powder.

Add ½ tsp (2 mL) spirulina for added antioxidants and protein.

Add either ground flaxseed or seed mixture to get more fiber, protein and omega-3 fats.

This recipe is a nice blend of fruits with the added liquid and vitamins from the romaine lettuce. It's a bit low in protein, but several super enhancers—including liquid or powder protein, flax, seed mixture and spirulina—can improve this. And it boasts an impressive list of phytochemicals and a delicious taste.

1 cup (250 mL)	pitted peach (5 oz/140 g)
¼ cup (60 mL)	blueberries (1¼ oz/35 g)
¼ cup (60 mL)	hulled strawberries (1 oz/30 g)
1 cup (250 mL)	peeled seeded honeydew melon (5 oz/140 g)
1 cup (250 mL)	packed romaine lettuce (1 oz/28 g)
2 tbsp (30 mL)	coconut water

1. Wash all produce well and cut into chunks.

2. Place all ingredients in blender and process until desired consistency.

Makes 1 serving (1 cup/250 mL/265 g)

Phytochemicals
ALA, alpha- and beta-carotene, anthocyanidin, caffeic acid, campesterol, cathechin, catechol, chlorogenic acid, cryptoxanthin, cyanidin, ellagic acid, eugenol, ferulic acid, flavonols, gallic acid, hydroxycinnamic acid, kaempferol, limonene, lutein, luteolin, lycopene, matairesinol, myricetin, oleanolic acid, pelargonidin, phytosterols, quercetin, rosmarinic acid, rutin, secoisolariciresinol, urosolic acid, zeaxanthin

100% Daily requirement

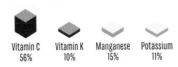

Vitamin C 56% Vitamin K 10% Manganese 15% Potassium 11%

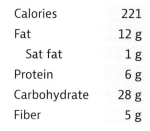

G'Day Down Under

This tasty treat is a truly unique blend of tasty superfoods — kiwi, coconut and macadamia nuts — now found on the continent Down Under. All nuts are chock full of essential nutrients and phytochemicals, and each brings its unique texture and taste to a recipe. When using nuts in the blender or food processor, it often works best to process them first to get a smoother consistency and not chunks.

Calories		221
Fat		12 g
Sat fat		1 g
Protein		6 g
Carbohydrate		28 g
Fiber		5 g

	1	peeled medium kiwifruit (2½ oz/70 g)
	1 cup (250 mL)	peach slices (about 1 medium) (5 oz/150 g)
	2 tbsp (30 mL)	macadamia nuts (½ oz/16 g)
	¼ cup (60 mL)	coconut water

1. Place nuts in blender and process to consistency of meal.

2. Cut kiwi in half and place in blender with peaches (leave skin on). Add coconut water.

3. Process until desired consistency.

Makes 1 serving (1½ cups/375 mL/295 g)

100% Daily requirement

Vitamin C	Folate	Vitamin K	Pantothenic Acid	Iron	Potassium
126%	19%	24%	13%	13%	13%

Phytochemicals
Anthocyanidin, cryptoxanthin, cyanidin, flavonols, lutein, lycopene, phytosterols, quercetin, zeaxanthin

177

Red Pepper Mango

Calories	122
Fat	1 g
Sat fat	0
Protein	2 g
Carbohydrate	31 g
Fiber	4 g

Super Enhancer Tip

If you'd like more protein, you can add ¼ cup (60 mL) Greek yogurt or 2 tbsp (30 mL) ground flaxseed.

The red pepper works very well in combination with fruits, and it's an excellent way to lower calories and increase both nutrients and phytochemicals in a juice or smoothie recipe. This recipe needed a touch more sweetness, so we added one date, which proved adequate. If you don't have dates, you can add honey or any other type of sweetener.

	½	pitted medium mango (4 oz/115 g)
	½ cup (125 mL)	seeded ribbed red bell pepper (1¼ oz/36 g)
	½ cup (125 mL)	frozen sour cherries (2 oz/60 g)
	1	date (¼ oz/7 g)
	2 tbsp (30 mL)	water

1. Wash all produce well.

2. Add all ingredients to blender and process until desired consistency.

Makes 1 serving (1 cup/250 mL/250 g)

Phytochemicals

ALA, alpha- and beta-carotene, anacardic acid, caffeic acid, campesterol, capsaicin, catechins, chlorogenic acid, cinnamic acid, cryptoxanthin, eugenol, gallic acid, hesperidin, kaempferol, limonene, lutein, mangiferin, naringenin, phytoene, phytofluene, phytosterols, proanthocyanidins, quercetin, rutin, tannins, zeaxanthin

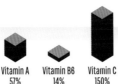

100% Daily requirement

Vitamin A	Vitamin B6	Vitamin C	Folate	Vitamin K	Potassium
57%	14%	150%	18%	10%	11%

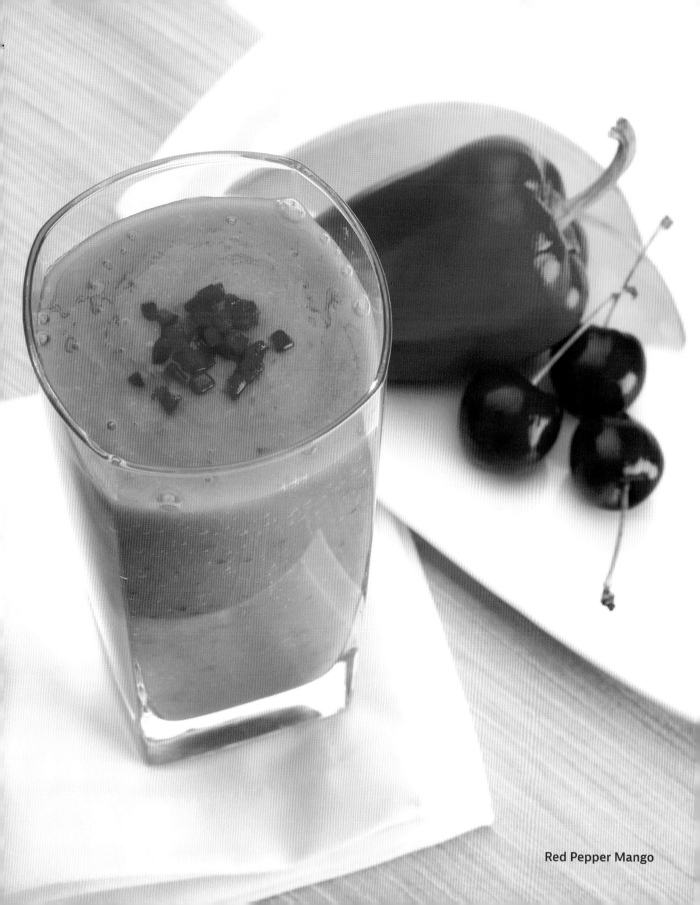

Red Pepper Mango

Easy Breezy

Calories	91
Fat	0
Sat fat	0
Protein	1 g
Carbohydrate	21 g
Fiber	10 g

Super Enhancer Tips

👍 Add 1 tbsp (15 mL) vanilla whey protein or fruit-flavored liquid protein for the extra protein to see you through to lunch.

👍 Boost fiber in this recipe with a tablespoon (15 mL) of seed mixture.

This light-tasting juice gives you an entire day's supply of vitamin C and numerous phytochemicals. For only three ingredients, you'll have a quick and healthful juice to grab and go. By adding a few super enhancers, you can also boost nutrition.

½ cup (125 mL)	peeled seeded papaya (3 oz/80 g)
2 cups (500 mL)	packed romaine lettuce (1¾ oz/50 g)
1 cup (250 mL)	peeled seeded honeydew melon (4 oz/115 g)

1. Wash all produce well.

2. Add all ingredients to blender and process until desired consistency.

Makes 1 serving (1 cup/250 mL/245 g)

Phytochemicals

ALA, alpha- and beta-carotene, caffeic acid, campesterol, cryptoxanthin, cucurbitacin, ferulic acid, flavonols, kaempferol, lutein, luteolin, lycopene, phytoene, phytofluene, phytosterols, tannins, zeaxanthin

Vitamin C
121%

Folate
11%

No minerals present at 10% level

100% Daily requirement

Pango Dessert

Many recipes call for peeling peaches, but the blender does a great job with the skin. If you'd like to serve this as a dessert, keep it in the refrigerator for half a day until it thickens, then add yogurt and top with whipped cream.

🍑	1 cup (250 mL)	pitted peach (5 oz/150 g)
🥭	¾ cup (175 mL)	pitted mango (4 oz/115 g)
🌿	1 cup (250 mL)	packed arugula (1 oz/28 g)
	¼ cup (60 mL)	almond milk

1. Wash all produce well.

2. Add all ingredients to blender and process until desired consistency.

Makes 1 serving (1½ cups/375 mL/350 g)

Calories	152
Fat	2 g
Sat fat	0
Protein	3 g
Carbohydrate	36 g
Fiber	5 g

Super Enhancer Tip

Spirulina works very well in this recipe, in which the strong flavors of arugula and mango provide cover for that bit of fishy flavor this nutrient-dense algae sometimes imparts. You'll be boosting protein and antioxidants significantly by adding it to the recipe.

Phytochemicals
ALA, alpha- and beta-carotene, anacardic acid, anthocyanidin, caffeic acid, catechins, cryptoxanthin, flavonols, gallic acid, glucosinolates, indoles, kaempferol, lutein, lycopene, mangiferin, phytosterols, quercetin, sulforaphane, tannins, zeaxanthin

100% Daily requirement

Vitamin A	Vitamin C	Folate	Vitamin K	Calcium	Potassium
46%	92%	19%	43%	11%	17%

Broccoberry Dew

Calories	89
Fat	1 g
Sat fat	0
Protein	2 g
Carbohydrate	22 g
Fiber	4 g

Super Enhancer Tip

This recipe works well with some nuts, and we especially like a few tablespoons (start with 2 tbsp/30 mL) of walnuts, although pistachios are nice, too. This will boost protein, fiber and phytochemicals, as well as enhance the flavor.

Sulforaphane is a tremendous phytochemical in the fight against cancer. In addition, it also is a potent anti-inflammatory and antimicrobial compound. All the brassica family vegetables contain this compound, but broccoli is an especially good source. The melon and blueberries add their own impressive list of nutrients and phyto-chemicals, and, most importantly, sweet and tart flavors to mask the broccoli.

	1 cup (250 mL)	peeled seeded honeydew melon (4 oz/125 g)
	½ cup (125 mL)	broccoli florets (1¼ oz/37 g)
	½ cup (125 mL)	blueberries (2 oz/60 g)
	1 tsp (5 mL)	honey

1. Wash all produce well.

2. Add all ingredients to blender and process until desired consistency.

Makes 1 serving (1 cup/250 mL/220 g)

Phytochemicals

Alpha and beta-carotene, caffeic acid, campesterol, catechin, chlorogenic acid, cryptoxanthin, cucurbitacin, cyanidin, ellagic acid, eugenol, ferulic acid, gallic acid, hydroxycinnamic acid, indole-3 carbinol, isorhamnetin, kaempferol, lignan, limonene, lutein, matairesinol, myricetin, oleanolic acid, phytosterols, quercetin, rosmarinic acid, rutin, sinigrin, sulforaphane, urosolic acid

100% Daily requirement

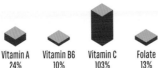

Vitamin A	Vitamin B6	Vitamin C	Folate	Vitamin K	Manganese	Potassium
24%	10%	103%	13%	20%	17%	12%

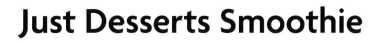

Just Desserts Smoothie

This tasty recipe is like a dessert, although its nutritional profile reflects eating double portions of vegetables. The pumpkin is our secret ingredient, and don't be shy about using it in canned form, as it's too easy and quick to pass up. Just make sure you buy pure pumpkin purée, not pie filling — the pie filling is sweetened. In moderate quantities, the strong flavor of pumpkin is easy to mask, as in this recipe. However, you may want to build on the flavor and include more pumpkin, since it's widely used in desserts. A few tablespoons (you could start with 2 tbsp/30 mL) of vanilla whey protein can transform this into a stick-to-your-ribs meal.

Calories		97
Fat		1 g
Sat fat		0
Protein		3 g
Carbohydrate		22 g
Fiber		5 g

Super Enhancer Tip

Add 2 tbsp (30 mL) vanilla whey protein powder for an additional 10 grams of protein.

	1	peeled medium kiwifruit (2½ oz/70 g)
	1	pitted medium peach (5 oz/140 g)
	½ cup (125 mL)	canned 100% pumpkin purée (4½ oz/125 g)
	¼ cup (60 mL)	soy milk
	1 piece (1 inch/2.5 cm)	gingerroot (¼ oz/6 g)
	1 slice (1 inch/2.5 cm)	lemon (1½ oz/40 g)
	1 tsp (5 mL)	honey

1. Wash all produce well. Peel ginger and lemon slice.

2. Add all ingredients to blender and process untils desired consistency.

Makes 2 servings (2 cups/500 mL/445 g)

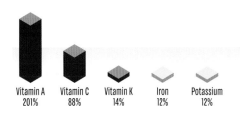

100% Daily requirement

Vitamin A	Vitamin C	Vitamin K	Iron	Potassium
201%	88%	14%	12%	12%

Phytochemicals
ALA, beta-carotene, anthocyanidin, caffeic acid, coumarin, cryptoxanthin, cyanidin, diosmin, ferulic acid, flavonols, gingerol, 6-dehydrogingerdione (dge), hesperidin, isorhamnetin, limonene, limonin, lutein, lycopene, phytosterols, quercetin, rutin, shogaols, zeaxanthin

Papayaberry Citrus

Calories	102
Fat	0
Sat fat	0
Protein	1 g
Carbohydrate	26 g
Fiber	4 g

Lemon and ginger work well together in recipes, and the phyto-chemicals they bring along are a dynamite combination. Studies show that one such phytochemical from the lemon, limonene, exhibits an incredible number of biologic effects. Some of these include antimicrobial, anti-inflammatory, immune enhancing and several anticancer effects.

	¾ cup (175 mL)	peeled seeded papaya (3½ oz/100 g)
	½ cup (125 mL)	blueberries (2½ oz/75 g)
	1 cup (250 mL)	packed romaine lettuce (1 oz/28 g)
	1 slice (½ inch/1 cm)	lemon (¾ oz/20 g)
	1 piece (1 inch/2.5 cm)	gingerroot (¼ oz/6 g)
	1	date (¼ oz/7 g)
	2 tbsp (30 mL)	coconut water

1. Wash all produce well; peel lemon and ginger.

2. Add all ingredients to blender and process until desired consistency.

Makes 1 serving (1 cup/250 mL/250 g)

Phytochemicals

ALA, alpha- and beta-carotene, caffeic acid, campesterol, catechin, chlorogenic acid, coumarin, cryptoxanthin, cyanidin, diosmin, ellagic acid, eugenol, ferullc acid, gallic acid, gingerol, 6-dehydrogingerdione (DGE), hesperidin, hydroxycinnamic acid, isorhamnetin, kaempferol, limonene, limonin, lutein, luteolin, lycopene, myricetin, oleanolic acid, phytoene, phytofluene, phytosterols, quercetin, rosmarinic acid, rutin, shogaols,tannins, urosolic acid, zeaxanthin

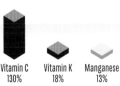

Vitamin C	Vitamin K	Manganese
130%	18%	13%

100% Daily requirement

Morning Dew

This recipe provides two great sources of lycopene in the red grapefruit and sweet red bell pepper. As you experiment with making your own juices and smoothies, remember to use red peppers frequently — their sweetness makes them taste like a fruit, but you'll know they're a vegetable by the nutrient profile!

Calories	175
Fat	5 g
Sat fat	0
Protein	3 g
Carbohydrate	33 g
Fiber	4 g

	5	red or pink grapefruit segments (4 oz/115 g)
	1 cup (250 mL)	peeled seeded honeydew melon (5 oz/150 g)
	½ cup (125 mL)	seeded ribbed red bell pepper (1½ oz/38 g)
	1 slice (½ inch/1 cm)	lemon (¾ oz/20 g)
	1 tbsp (15 mL)	walnuts (¼ oz/8 g)
	1	date (¼ oz/7 g)

1. Wash all produce well and peel lemon slice.

2. Add all ingredients to blender and process until desired consistency.

Makes 1 serving (1 cup/250 mL/315 g)

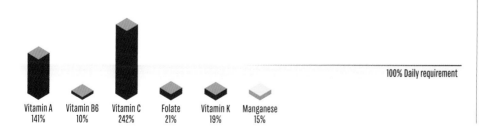

100% Daily requirement

Vitamin A	Vitamin B6	Vitamin C	Folate	Vitamin K	Manganese
141%	10%	242%	21%	19%	15%

Phytochemicals
ALA, alpha- and beta-carotene, caffeic acid, campesterol, capsaicin, chlorogenic acid, cinnamic acid, coumarin, cryptoxanthin, cucurbitacin, ellagic acid, eugenol, ferulic acid, hesperetin, hesperidin, isorhamnetin, limonene, lutein, lycopene, myricetin, phytoene, phytofluene, phytosterols, quercetin, zeaxanthin

Tofuberry Broccoli

Calories	156
Fat	2 g
Sat fat	0
Protein	8 g
Carbohydrate	31 g
Fiber	6 g

For those who don't care for tofu, an easy substitution is yogurt, especially Greek yogurt, which is thicker than regular yogurt. You won't get the isoflavones and phytosterols, but you'll pick up the probiotics. Remember that if you prefer a slushy consistency, use either frozen blueberries or add several ice cubes. We found that most of these blended treats did well with even floating ice cubes to keep them cold as we enjoyed sipping on them.

	½ cup (125 mL)	blueberries (2½ oz/75 g)
	½	cored medium apple (4 oz/112 g)
	½ cup (125 mL)	broccoli florets (1½ oz/38 g)
	½ cup (125 mL)	extra-firm silken tofu (2½ oz/80 g)
	¼ cup (60 mL)	water

1. Wash all produce well.

2. Add all ingredients to blender and process until desired consistency.

Makes 1 serving (1½ cups/375 mL/365 g)

Phytochemicals

Alpha- and beta carotene, caffeic acid, cathechins, chlorogenic acid, cryptoxanthin, cyanidin, ellagic acid, eugenol, ferulic acid, gallic acid, hydroxycinnamic acid, indole-3-carbinol, isorhamnetin, kaempferol, lignan, limonene, lutein, matairesinol, myricetin, oleanolic acid, phytosterols, procyanidins, quercetin, rosmarinic acid, rutin, sinigrin, sulforaphane, urosolic acid

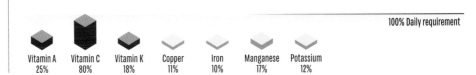

100% Daily requirement

Vitamin A	Vitamin C	Vitamin K	Copper	Iron	Manganese	Potassium
25%	80%	18%	11%	10%	17%	12%

Strawberry Dew

This great recipe gets its low calorie and carbohydrate levels from the addition of mushrooms. The mushrooms also bring in nutrients not usually found in most fruits and vegetables, which include several B vitamins and the mineral selenium. The latter is important in an antioxidant enzyme system in the body, so it can help protect against several chronic diseases.

🍓	¾ cup (175 mL)	hulled strawberries (3½ oz/100 g)
🍈	1 cup (250 mL)	peeled seeded honeydew melon (5 oz/150 g)
🍄	1 cup (125 mL)	mushrooms (1½ oz/44 g)
	1 tbsp (15 mL)	vanilla whey protein powder

1. Wash all produce well.

2. Add all ingredients to blender and process until desired consistency.

Makes 1 serving (1¼ cups/300 mL/295 g)

Calories	96
Fat	1 g
Sat fat	0
Protein	3 g
Carbohydrate	23 g
Fiber	4 g

Super Enhancer Tip

👍 Add ground flaxseed for extra protein, omega-3 fats and fiber.

Phytochemicals
Alpha- and beta-carotene, beta-glucans, caffeic acid, campesterol, catechin, catechol, chlorogenic acid, cryptoxanthin, cucurbitacin, ellagic acid, ferulic acid, gallic acid, kaempferol, lutein, matairesinol, pelargonidin, phytosterols, secoisolariciresinol, zeaxanthin

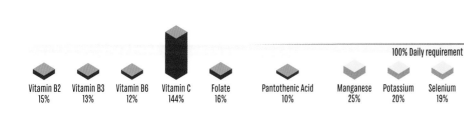

| Vitamin B2 15% | Vitamin B3 13% | Vitamin B6 12% | Vitamin C 144% | Folate 16% | Pantothenic Acid 10% | Manganese 25% | Potassium 20% | Selenium 19% |

100% Daily requirement

Asian Delight

Calories	133
Fat	1 g
Sat fat	0
Protein	3 g
Carbohydrate	32 g
Fiber	11 g

The Asian pear is shaped like an apple, but it tastes decidedly like a pear. It originated in various countries in Asia and is often referred to as a Japanese, Chinese or Korean pear. Like other pears, it's high in fiber and anthocyanidins — a group of phytochemicals that act as antioxidants, and some studies have shown they protect oral health. Friedelin is another phytochemical in pears with anti-inflammatory effects. The Asian pear is also higher in water content, which makes it perfect for juicing, although it is sometimes more expensive.

	¾ cup (175 mL)	raspberries (3½ oz/100 g)
	1 cup (250 ml)	packed spinach (¾ oz/20 g)
	½ cup (125 mL)	baby carrots (2 oz/60 g)
	½	cored medium Asian pear (3 oz/85 g)
	¼ cup (60 ml)	coconut water

1. Wash all produce well.

2. Add all ingredients to blender and process until desired consistency.

Makes 1 serving (1½ cups/375 mL/340 g)

Phytochemicals

ALA alpha- and beta carotene, anthocyanidins, bergapten, caffeic acid, campesterol, catechin, catechol, chlorogenic acid, chlorophyll, coumarin, coumestrol, cryptoxanthin, cucurbitacin, ellagic acid, ferulic acid, friedelin, gallic acid, geraniol, kaempferol, lupeol, lutein, luteolin, lycopene, matairesinol, pelargonidin, phytofluene, phytosterols, quercetin, rutin, secoisolariciresinol, urosolic acid, zeaxanthin

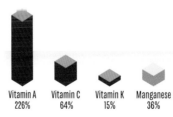

100% Daily requirement

Vitamin A	Vitamin C	Vitamin K	Manganese
226%	64%	15%	36%

Peach Pom Verde

Collard greens are one of the most nutrient-dense of the leafy green vegetables. Surprisingly, they don't yield a large amount of juice, so they work very well in the blender, where you'll get the fiber, too. This recipe uses the pomegranate seeds only, which makes for a sweeter juice, rather than merely peeling a pomegranate.

Calories	113
Fat	1 g
Sat fat	0
Protein	2 g
Carbohydrate	29 g
Fiber	6 g

🍈	¼ cup (60 mL)	pomegranate seeds (1½ oz/40 g)
🍑	½	pitted medium peach (2 oz/52 g)
🍎	½	cored large Red Delicious apple (3½ oz/100 g)
🌿	1 cup (250 mL)	packed chopped collard greens (1 oz/25 g)

1. Wash all produce well.

2. Add all ingredients to blender and process until desire consistency.

Makes 1 serving (1 cup/250 mL/220 g)

Vitamin A	Vitamin C	Folate	Vitamin K	Potassium
37%	35%	14%	168%	10%

100% Daily requirement

Phytochemicals
ALA, anthocyanidins, caffeic acid, carotenoids, catechins, chlorogenic acid, cyanidin, ellagic acid, flavonols, isoquercetin, isorhamnetin, lutein, lycopene, phytosterols, procyanidins, punicalagins, quercetin, ursolic acid

Morning Greenery

Calories	100
Fat	1 g
Sat fat	0
Protein	3 g
Carbohydrate	22 g
Fiber	3 g

Super Enhancer Tips

 Add 2 tbsp (30 mL) vanilla whey protein powder.

Add 2 tbsp (30 mL) ground flaxseed for more protein and extra fiber and omega-2 fats.

If your local store does not carry kefir, you can substitute yogurt and maintain the probiotic benefit of this smoothie. This Is another lower-calorie beverage, so you can add a protein source, such as vanilla whey protein. You can also ground flaxseed.

	2 cups (500 mL)	peeled seeded honeydew melon (10 oz/300 g)
	1	pitted small nectarine (3¼ oz/92 g)
	2 cups (500 mL)	packed chopped collard greens (2 oz/60 g)
	¼ cup (60 mL)	almond milk
	1 tbsp (15 mL)	kefir cheese (labne) (½ oz/14 g)

1. Wash all produce well.

2. Add all ingredients to blender and process until desired consistency.

Makes 2 servings (2 cups/500 mL/525 g)

Phytochemicals

ALA, alpha- and beta-carotene, anthocyanidin, caffeic acid, campesterol, cryptoxanthin, cucurbitacin, ferulic acid, flavonols, lutein, lycopene, phytosterols, quercetin, zeaxanthin

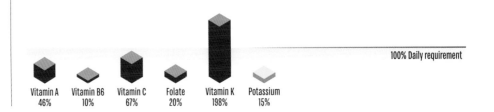

Vitamin A	Vitamin B6	Vitamin C	Folate	Vitamin K	Potassium
46%	10%	67%	20%	198%	15%

100% Daily requirement

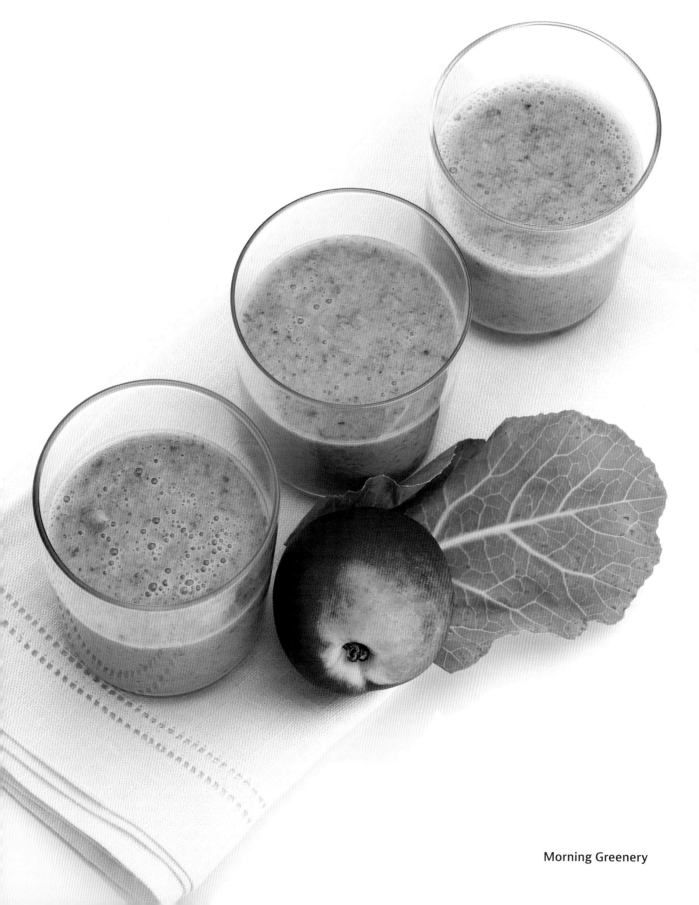

Morning Greenery

Pomberry Citrus

Calories	130
Fat	1 g
Sat fat	0
Protein	3 g
Carbohydrate	32 g
Fiber	6 g

Arugula and blueberries meld well together, and this recipe adds the antioxidant power of the orange and pomegranate. If you try your hand at growing your own arugula, make sure to invest in a salad spinner. This handy kitchen gadget removes all debris and produces a clean green!

	¼ cup (60 mL)	pomegranate seeds (1½ oz/40 g)
	½ peeled	medium orange (3½ oz/100 g)
	1 cup (250 mL)	packed arugula (1 oz/28 g)
	½ cup (125 mL)	blueberries (2½ oz/75 g)

1. Wash all produce well.

2. Add all ingredients to blender and process until desired consistency.

Makes 1 serving (1 cup/250 mL/240 g)

Phytochemicals

ALA, alpha- and beta-carotene, caffeic acid, cathechins, chlorogenic acid, cryptoxanthin, coumarin, cyanidin, ellagic acid, eugenol, ferulic acid, gallic acid, glucosinolates, hydroxycinnamic acid, indoles, limonene, lutein, myricetin, oleanolic acid, phytoene, phytofluene, phytosterols, punicalagins, quercetin, rosmarinic acid, rutin, sulforaphane, urosolic acid, zeaxanthin

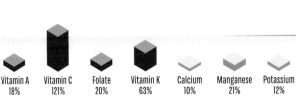

Vitamin A	Vitamin C	Folate	Vitamin K	Calcium	Manganese	Potassium
18%	121%	20%	63%	10%	21%	12%

100% Daily requirement

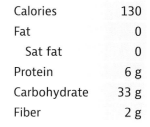

Gingersnap

This was one of our favorite recipes, and we made a double batch a few days after developing it! The ginger enlivens the other ingredients and the vanilla whey protein mellows out the flavor, in addition to adding protein. Of course, the nutritional analysis also made us love this one, providing a day's supply of vitamins A and C and a long list of phytochemicals.

	½	cored medium Bosc pear (3½ oz/100 g)
	½	peeled medium orange (3½ oz/100 g)
1 piece (¾ inch/2 cm)		gingerroot (⅛ oz/4 g)
¼ cup (60 mL)		coconut water
1 tbsp (15 mL)		vanilla whey protein powder

1. Wash all produce well and peel ginger.

2. Add all ingredients to blender and process until desired consistency.

Makes 1 serving (1½ cups/325 mL/300 g)

Calories	130
Fat	0
Sat fat	0
Protein	6 g
Carbohydrate	33 g
Fiber	2 g

100% Daily requirement

Vitamin A 178% Vitamin C 112% Folate 10%   No minerals present at 10% level

Phytochemicals
ALA, alpha- and beta-carotene, anthocyanidins, bergapten, caffeic acid, campesterol, chlorogenic acid, coumarin, cryptoxanthin,cyanidin, ferulic acid,friedelin, geraniol, gingerol, 6-dehydrogingerdione (DGE), limonene, lupeol, lutein, lycopene, phytoene, phytofluene, phytosterols, shogaols,secoisolariciresinol, ursolic acid, zeaxanthin

Jasmine Power Blend

Calories	146
Fat	1 g
Sat fat	0
Protein	3 g
Carbohydrate	35 g
Fiber	8 g

This beverage simply bursts with antioxidant muscle. And if that weren't enough, the essential nutrients are also off the charts. The pomegranate and raspberries give a magnificent color and terrific flavor, while the jasmine green tea provides liquid and also key phytochemicals.

	¼ cup (50 mL)	pomegranate seeds (1½ oz/40 g)
	1	peeled medium kiwifruit (2 oz/54 g)
	5	red or pink grapefruit segments (3 oz/115 g)
	½ cup (125 mL)	raspberries (2 oz/55 g)
	½ cup (125 mL)	mushrooms (1½ oz/44 g)
	¼ cup (60 mL)	jasmine tea

1. Wash all produce well.

2. Add all ingredients to blender and process until desired consistency.

Makes 1 serving (1¾ cups/425 mL/370 g)

Phytochemicals
ALA, alpha- and beta-carotene, anthocyanidins, beta-glucans, caffeic acid, campesterol, coumarin, cryptoxanthin, cyanidins, ellagic acid, ferulic acid, hesperetin, hesperidin, isorhamnetin, limonene, lutein, pelargonidin, phytoene, phytofluene, quercetin, zeaxanthin

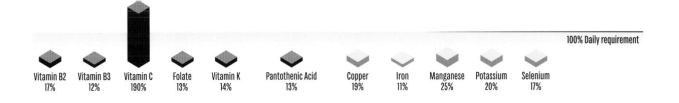

| Vitamin B2 17% | Vitamin B3 12% | Vitamin C 190% | Folate 13% | Vitamin K 14% | Pantothenic Acid 13% | Copper 19% | Iron 11% | Manganese 25% | Potassium 20% | Selenium 17% | 100% Daily requirement |

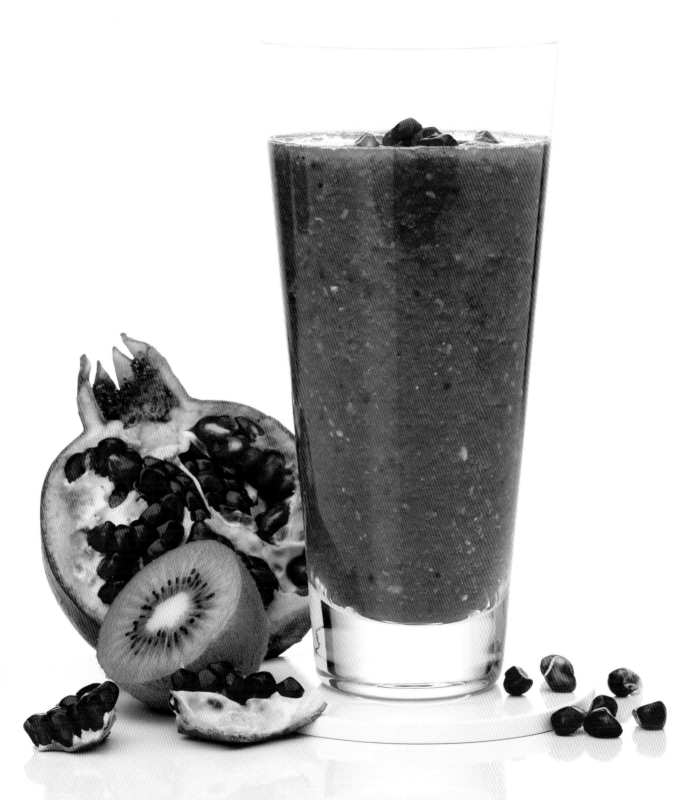

Jasmine Power Blend

Broccoberry Date

Calories	87
Fat	1 g
Sat fat	0
Protein	5 g
Carbohydrate	21 g
Fiber	6 g

The only two produce items in this recipe are the berries and broccoli. The latter provides an interesting texture, and the addition of the seed mixture makes this beverage thicken up in a few hours in the refrigerator. If you need to thin it down later, you can add any type of milk or even more coconut water.

🍓	¾ cup (175 mL)	hulled strawberries (3½ oz/100 g)
🥦	¾ cup (175 mL)	broccoli florets (2 oz/58 g)
	2 tbsp (30 mL)	coconut water
	2	dates (½ oz/14 g each)
	½ tbsp (7 mL)	seed mix

1. Wash all produce well.

2. Add all ingredients to blender and process until desired consistency.

Makes 1 serving (1 cup/250 mL/200 g)

Phytochemicals
ALA, caffeic acid, catechins, catechol, chlorogenic acid, ellagic acid, ferulic acid, gallic acid, indole-3-carbinol, isorhamnetin, kaempferol, lignan, lutein, matairesinol, myricetin, pelargonidin, phytosterols, quercetin, secoisolariciresinol, sinigrin, sulforaphane, zeaxanthin

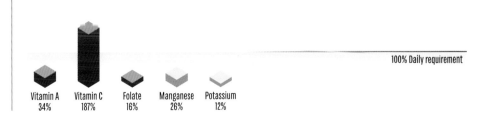

100% Daily requirement

Vitamin A	Vitamin C	Folate	Manganese	Potassium
34%	187%	16%	26%	12%

Double Berry Veggie

This recipe is low in calories and high in everything else that counts. Check the phytochemical list — it's a veritable who's who of stars. One of these compounds, isorhamnetin, is not too familiar to most, but it's worth getting to know about it. The studies show antioxidant, anti-inflammatory and antibacterial effects. In addition, it seems to protect the liver against potential toxins. The flavors combine to form a pleasantly sweet beverage, and the lime gives it a tart kick.

	⅓ cup (75 mL)	blackberries (1¾ oz/48 g)
	¼ cup (60 mL)	baby carrots (2 oz/60 g)
	½ cup (125 mL)	hulled strawberries (2¼ oz/65 g)
	½ cup (125 mL)	seeded ribbed red bell pepper (2 oz/55 g)
	1 slice (½ inch/1 cm)	lime (¾ oz/22 g)

1. Wash all produce well and peel lime slice.

2. Add all ingredients to blender and process until desired consistency.

Makes 1 serving (1 cup/250 mL/260 g)

Calories		85
Fat		1 g
Sat fat		0
Protein		3 g
Carbohydrate		19 g
Fiber		6 g

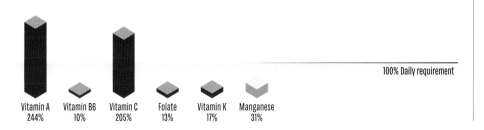

100% Daily requirement

Vitamin A	Vitamin B6	Vitamin C	Folate	Vitamin K	Manganese
244%	10%	205%	13%	17%	31%

Phytochemicals
ALA, alpha- and beta-carotene, bergapten, caffeic acid, campesterol, capsaicin, catechin, catechol, chlorogenic acid, cinnamic acid, coumarin, cryptoxanthin, cyanidin, ellagic acid, eugenol, ferulic acid, gallic acid, geraniol, hesperidin, isorhamnetin, kaempferol, lignans, limonene, lupeol, lutein, luteolin, lycopene, matairesinol, pelargonidin, phenolic acids, phytoene, phytofluene, phytosterols, quercetin, secoisolariciresinol, stilbenoids, tannins, zeaxanthin

Pumpkinberry Tart

Calories	140
Fat	3 g
Sat fat	0
Protein	5 g
Carbohydrate	28 g
Fiber	10 g

This delicious recipe will give you almost four times the vitamin A you need in a day, as well as many other essential nutrients. The iron level, for example, is surprisingly high for a fruit and vegetable juice, which is important because many women and children don't get an adequate amount every day.

🍓	¾ cup (175 mL)	hulled strawberries (3½ oz/100 g)
🍒	¼ cup (60 mL)	frozen tart cherries (1 oz/30 g)
🎃	½ cup (125 mL)	canned 100% pumpkin (4 oz/120 g)
🍋	1 slice (½ inch/1 cm)	lemon (¾ oz/20 g)
	6 tbsp (90 mL)	coconut water
	1 tbsp (15 mL)	ground flaxseed (¼ oz/7g)
	1 tsp (5 mL)	honey

1. Wash all produce well; peel and seed lemon slice.

2. Add all ingredients to blender and process until desired consistency.

Makes 1 serving (1½ cups/375 mL/370 g)

Phytochemicals
ALA, beta-carotene, caffeic acid, catechins, catechol, chlorogenic acid, coumarin, diosmin, ellagic acid, ferulic acid, gallic acid, hesperidin, kaempferol, isorhamnetin, limonene, limonin, lutein, matairesinol, naringenin, pelargonidin, phytosterols, proanthocyanidins, rutin, secoisolariciresinol, zeaxanthin

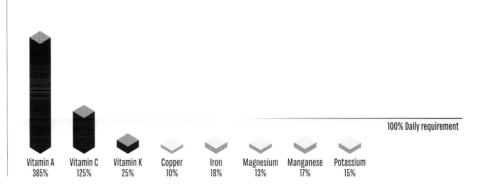

Vitamin A	Vitamin C	Vitamin K	Copper	Iron	Magnesium	Manganese	Potassium
385%	125%	25%	10%	18%	13%	17%	15%

100% Daily requirement

Fuzzy Pom

Pomegranate can be blended with or without the membranes as well as the seeds, but make sure it's ripe and that you remove the peel and as much of the pith as possible, which is not quite as time-consuming as extracting only the seeds. Some of our tasters did not care for pomegranate recipes that did not use only seeds, but we liked them. The membranes impart a tart astringency, but it can be masked fairly well if you don't purchase the pricey seeds alone.

	½	small pomegranate (3½ oz/100 g)
	2	pitted medium apricots (3½ oz/100 g)
	½ cup (125 mL)	baby carrots (1¾ oz/52 g)
	½	cored medium Bartlett pear (3 oz/80 g)
	1 cup (150 mL)	almond milk
	2 tsp (10 mL)	honey

1. Wash all produce well. Using a paring knife, remove skin and excess pith from pomegranate.

2. Add all ingredients to blender and process until desired consistency.

Makes 2 servings (2 cups/500 mL/560 g)

Calories	125
Fat	3 g
Sat fat	0
Protein	2 g
Carbohydrate	25 g
Fiber	5 g

Phytochemicals
ALA, alpha- and beta-carotene, anthocyanidins, bergapten, caffeic acid, campesterol, chlorogenic acid, coumarin, cryptoxanthin, cyanidin, ellagic acid, ferulic acid,friedelin, geraniol, isoquercetin, lupeol, lutein, luteolin, lycopene, phytofluene, phytosterols, punicalagins, quercetin, secoisolariciresinol, ursolic acid

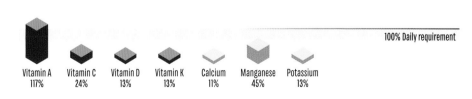

Vitamin A 117%	Vitamin C 24%	Vitamin D 13%	Vitamin K 13%	Calcium 11%	Manganese 45%	Potassium 13%

100% Daily requirement

Morning Chocoblast

Calories	152
Fat	2 g
Sat fat	0
Protein	11 g
Carbohydrate	23 g
Fiber	5 g

Wake yourself up with this delicious smoothie that brings the flavors of the sweet pear and velvety dark chocolate to a morning staple. The whey protein and beans complete the nutritional package, and they also make this a filling beverage. If you're using canned beans, be sure to rinse them well.

	¼ cup (60 mL)	black beans (1½ oz/42 g)
	½	cored medium Bartlett pear (2½ oz/80 g)
	½ cup (125 mL)	brewed dark-roast coffee
	1 tbsp (15 mL)	vanilla whey protein powder
	1 tbsp (15 mL)	dark unsweetened cocoa powder

Add all ingredients to blender and process until desired consistency.

Makes 1 serving (1 cup/250 mL/240 g)

Phytochemicals
ALA, anthocyanidins, caffeic acid, campesterol, catechins, chlorogenic acid, coumarin, cyanidin, eugenol, ferulic acid, friedelin, gallic acid, flavonols, lutein, hytosterols,proanthocyanidins, squalene, tannins, theaflavins, trigonelline, ursolic acid

No vitamins or minerals present at 10% level

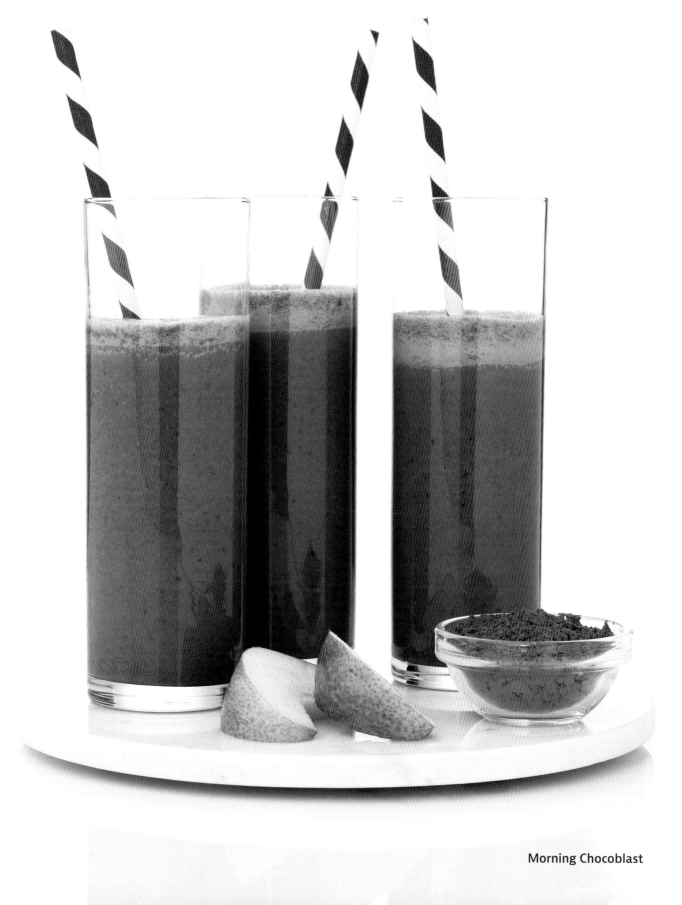

Morning Chocoblast

Pearberry Tofu

Calories	125
Fat	2 g
Sat fat	0
Protein	4 g
Carbohydrate	24 g
Fiber	6 g

Super Enhancer Tip

Add 1 tbsp (15 mL) vanilla whey protein powder or fruit-flavored liquid protein to boost protein.

This sweet treat includes two supervegetables, but you wouldn't know it from the luscious flavor. If you freeze the strawberries and pear, you'll have a delicious slushy. The tofu gives this treat some protein, so it's a great meal on the run.

	¾ cup (175 mL)	hulled strawberries (3½ oz/100 g)
	⅓	seeded ribbed large red bell pepper (2 oz/32 g)
	2 tbsp (30 mL)	silken tofu (2 oz/30 g)
	¼ cup (60 mL)	almond milk
	½ cup (125 mL)	cored Asian pear (1½ oz/45 g)
	1	date (¼ oz/7 g)
	1 cup (250 mL)	chopped cabbage (2¼ oz/65 g)

1. Wash all produce well.

2. Add red pepper, tofu, almond milk, strawberries, pear and date to blender and process.

3. Add cabbage last, adding more liquid if needed.

Makes 1 serving (1½ cups/375 mL/340 g)

Phytochemicals

ALA, alpha-carotene, anthocyanidins, caffeic acid, campesterol, capsaicin, cathechins, catechol, chlorogenic acid, cinnamic acid, cryptoxanthin, cyanidins, ellagic acid, eugenol, ferulic acid, friedelin, gallic acid, hesperidin, isoflavones, indole-3-carbinol, kaempferol, lignans, limonene, lutein, lycopene, matairesinol, pelargonidin, phytoene, phytofluene, phytosterols, quercetin, secoisolariciresinol, sinigrin, ursolic acid, zeaxanthin

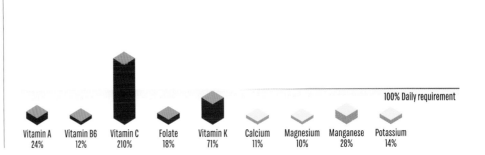

Vitamin A	Vitamin B6	Vitamin C	Folate	Vitamin K	Calcium	Magnesium	Manganese	Potassium
24%	12%	210%	18%	71%	11%	10%	28%	14%

100% Daily requirement

Sweet Berry Greens

Wheatgrass has become very popular, especially as a juicing ingredient, although its use dates back to the early 1930s. It contains similar nutrients as leafy greens and is high in phytochemicals. Along with asparagus, it keeps the calories and carbs low in this recipe.

Wheatgrass can be grown in soil or water, and since it's used raw in juicing, it could be contaminated with microbes. Women who are pregnant or breastfeeding should avoid it. People who have celiac disease should also avoid wheatgrass.

	2	stalks asparagus (½ oz/18 g)
	¾ cup (175 mL)	hulled strawberries (5 oz/110 g)
	¼	peeled large orange (2 oz/62 g)
	¼ cup (60 mL)	wheatgrass (⅛ oz/4 g)
	6 tbsp (90 mL)	water

1. Wash all produce well. Break off lower portion of asparagus stalks.

2. Add all ingredients to blender and process until desired consistency.

Makes 1 serving (1 cup/250 mL/285 g)

Calories	69
Fat	0
Sat fat	2 g
Protein	3 g
Carbohydrate	17 g
Fiber	4 g

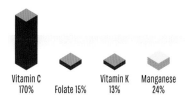

100% Daily requirement

Vitamin C 170% Folate 15% Vitamin K 13% Manganese 24%

Phytochemicals
ALA, alpha- and beta-carotene, caffeic acid, catechins, catechol, chlorogenic acid, chlorophyll, coumarin, cryptoxanthin, diosgenin, ellagic acid, ferulic acid, gallic acid, inositol, kaempferol, limonene, lutein, matairesinol, pelargonidin, oleic acid, phenols, phytoene, phytofluene, phytosterols, saponin, secoisolariciresinol, zeaxanthin

Avocadowow

Calories	215
Fat	15 g
Sat fat	2 g
Protein	6 g
Carbohydrate	19 g
Fiber	9 g

Kefir is a fermented milk drink that contains probiotics and the healthy nutrients from the milk. Labne is a cheese made from kefir and has a thicker consistency. This delicious recipe contains abundant nutrients, phytochemicals and healthy probiotics. The avocado is high in fat from monounsaturated fatty acids, so it's good for your heart. The beans add to that benefit by providing soluble fiber, which has been shown to lower cholesterol levels.

	1	peeled pitted medium avocado (3 oz/90 g)
	½	peeled medium cucumber (5 oz/135 g)
	2 tbsp (30 ml)	chopped onion (½ oz/14 g)
	¼ cup (60 mL)	water
	2 tbsp (30 mL)	kefir cheese (labne) (1 oz/30 g)
	2 tbsp (30 mL)	black beans (1 oz/30 g)
	¼ tsp (5 mL)	ground cumin
	1 tbsp (15 mL)	freshly squeezed lemon juice
		Pinch of salt

1. Add water and kefir to blender, then add vegetables and beans and blend until desired consistency.

2. Stir in cumin, lemon juice and salt after blending.

Makes 1 serving (1¼ cups/300 mL/255 g)

Phytochemicals
Apigenin, beta-sitosterol, cryptoxanthin, lutein, eugenol, inositol hexaphosphate, limonene luteolin, quercetin, saponins, tartaric acid

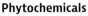

100% Daily requirement

Vitamin B6 12% · Vitamin C 31% · Folate 19% · Vitamin K 24% · Pantothenic Acid 13% · Potassium 15%

Pizza Time

This is a fun recipe that several members of our tasting panel said they would enjoy as a beverage. However, a few others suggested it might be better as a hot soup or sauce for pasta and other grains. Either way, it's loaded with phytochemicals, notably from the presence of garlic, onions and oregano. The tomato and carrots round out the nutrient profile with vitamins A and C.

	Calories	174
	Fat	2 g
	Sat fat	0
	Protein	8 g
	Carbohydrate	33 g
	Fiber	3 g

	⅓	large carrot (1¼ oz/35 g)
	½ cup (125 mL)	medium tomato (1 medium, 3 ½ oz/104 g)
	½ cup (125 mL)	chickpeas (2¾ oz/80 g)
	2 tbsp (30 mL)	water
	¼	medium onion (2 oz/58 g)
	1	clove garlic
	2 tbsp (30 mL)	fresh oregano (2 oz/58 g)

1. Place carrot, tomato, chickpeas and water in blender and process.

2. Add onion, garlic and oregano and pulse (use the stop/start toggle switch several times) until desired consistency.

Makes 2 servings (1½ cups/375 mL/370 g)

Super Enhancer Tip

Add 2 tbsp (30 mL) kefir cheese (labne) for a cheesy flavor and a shot of probiotics.

Phytochemicals
ALA, allicin, alpha- and beta-carotene, anthocyanin, apigenin, bergapten, caffeic acid, campesterol, catechol, chlorogenic acid, chlorophyll, cinnamic acid, coumarin, cryptoxanthin, diallyl sulfide, eugenol, ferulic acid, geraniol, glucosinolates, isorhamnetin, kaempferol, limonene, lupeol, luteolin, lycopene, naringenin, oleanolic acid, phytoene, phytofluene, phytosterols, quercetin, rosmarinic acid, rutin, saponins, secoisolariciresinol, squalene, tannins, urosolic acid, zeaxanthin

100% Daily requirement

Vitamin A	Vitamin C	Copper
123%	43%	11%

Chick V3

Calories	137
Fat	2 g
Sat fat	0
Protein	7 g
Carbohydrate	25 g
Fiber	3 g

Super Enhancer Tip

Add a teaspoon (5 mL) of spirulina powder to enhance the protein and antioxidant power of this savory beverage.

This savory beverage is another smoothie that you may prefer to use as a soup or sauce. It's high powered by the healthy dose of rosemary, which contains unique phytochemicals. In fact, a recent study reported that this aromatic herb was especially protective of brain tissue, with one of the researchers remarking that it "exerted a drug-like effect, but only when needed."

	⅓	large carrot (1¼ oz/35 g)
	½ cup (125 mL)	tomato (1 medium, 3½ oz/104 g)
	6 tbsp (90 ml)	water
	½ cup (125 mL)	chickpeas (2¼ oz/70 g)
	½ cup (125 mL)	broccoli florets (1½ oz/44 g)
	2 tbsp (30 ml)	fresh rosemary (⅛ oz/4 g)

1. Place carrot, tomato and water in blender and process.

2. Add chickpeas, broccoli and rosemary and pulse (use the stop/start toggle switch several times) until desired consistency.

Makes 1 serving (1¼ cups/300 mL/315 g)

Phytochemicals

ALA, alpha- and beta-carotene, apigenin, bergapten, caffeic acid, campesterol, carnasole, chlorogenic acid, chlorophyll, coumarin, cryptoxanthin, diosmin, eugenol, ferulic acid, geraniol, hesperidin, indole-3-carbinol, isorhamnetin, kaempferol, lignan, limonene, lupeol, lutein, luteolin, lycopene, matairesinol, myricetin, naringenin, phytoene, phytofluene, phytosterols, quercetin, rosemarinol, rutin, secoisolariciresinol, sinigrin, squalene, sulforaphane, ursolic acid, zeaxanthin

100% Daily requirement

Vitamin A	Vitamin C	Folate	Copper	Manganese
127%	98%	15%	10%	32%

Mediterranean Veggie

This Middle Eastern–inspired recipe can double as a savory beverage, perhaps for lunch, and a great-tasting soup when heated. You can use powdered turmeric or fresh ground root, if available. The important phytochemicals in this amazing herb will be present in both forms. The majority of our tasting panel did not like a higher amount, so we settled on ½ tsp (2 mL). You can try increasing it for additional antioxidant and anti-inflammatory potency. Proceed slowly, however, and increase by only another fourth, as it has a bitter flavor.

Calories	115
Fat	1 g
Sat fat	0
Protein	8 g
Carbohydrate	17 g
Fiber	1 g

	¾ cup (175 mL)	tomato (1 medium, 4 oz/124 g)
	½ cup (125 mL)	chickpeas (2½ oz/78 g)
	2 cups (500 mL)	packed romaine lettuce (2 oz/55 g)
	¼	medium onion (2 oz/58 g)
	1 slice (½ inch/1 cm)	lemon (¾ oz/20 g)
	½ cup (125 mL)	nonfat Greek yogurt (4 oz/115 g)
	¼ cup (60 mL)	water
	½ tsp (2 mL)	ground turmeric
	½ tsp (2 mL)	ground cumin

1. Wash all produce well. Remove rind and seeds from lemon.

2. Add all ingredients to blender and pulse (use the stop/start toggle switch several times) until desired consistency.

Makes 2 servings (2 cups/500 mL/510 g)

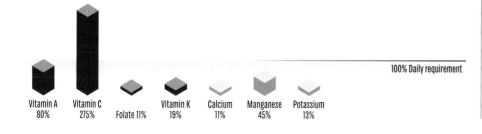

100% Daily requirement

Vitamin A 80% · Vitamin C 275% · Folate 11% · Vitamin K 19% · Calcium 11% · Manganese 45% · Potassium 13%

Phytochemicals
ALA, anthocyanin, caffeic acid, campesterol, chlorogenic acid, chlorophyll, cinnamic acid, coumarin, curcumin, diosmin, eugenol, ferulic acid, glucosinolates, hesperidin, isorhamnetin, kaempferol, limonene, limonin, lutein, luteolin, lycopene, naringenin, oleanolic acid, phytoene, phytofluene, phytosterols, quercetin, rutin, saponins, squalene, zeaxanthin

Abruzzi Fazu

Calories	166
Fat	1 g
Sat fat	0
Protein	10 g
Carbohydrate	31 g
Fiber	11 g

This is another savory beverage you can also use as a soup when heated. You can tell from the nutrient profile that it's a meal all by itself, even though the calorie level is quite low, but we also used it as an elegant sauce for a pasta and chicken entrée.

As a beverage, you can even double the amount of lemon. And if pecorino cheese isn't available, you can substitute grated Parmesan. The pecorino comes from sheep's milk, and it has a deeper and bolder flavor than Parmesan.

	½ cup (125 mL)	red kidney beans (4½ oz/130 g)
	2 cups (500 mL)	packed baby spinach (2 oz/52 g)
	¼	Vidalia onion (2 oz/58 g)
	1	clove garlic
	½ cup (125 mL)	seeded ribbed red bell pepper (2 oz/60 g)
	¼ cup (60 mL)	seeded ribbed green bell pepper (1½ oz/46 g)
	¼ cup (60 mL)	fresh basil leaves (¼ oz/6 g)
	1 tsp (5 mL)	freshly grated pecorino Romano cheese
	2 tbsp (30 mL)	water

1. Wash all produce well.

2. Add all ingredients to blender and process until desired consistency.

Makes 1 serving (1 1/2 cups/375 mL/300 g)

Phytochemicals
ALA, allicin, alpha-carotene, anthocyanin, caffeic acid, campesterol, capsaicin, chlorogenic acid, chlorophyll, cinnamic acid, coumestrol, cryptoxanthin, diallyl sulfide, eugenol, geraniol, glucosinolates, hesperidin, isorhamnetin, kaempferol, limonene, lutein, oleanolic acid, phytoene, phytofluene, phytosterols, quercetin, rutin, saponin, zeaxanthin

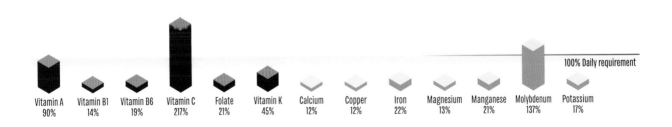

Vitamin A	Vitamin B1	Vitamin B6	Vitamin C	Folate	Vitamin K	Calcium	Copper	Iron	Magnesium	Manganese	Molybdenum	Potassium
90%	14%	19%	217%	21%	45%	12%	12%	22%	13%	21%	137%	17%

100% Daily requirement

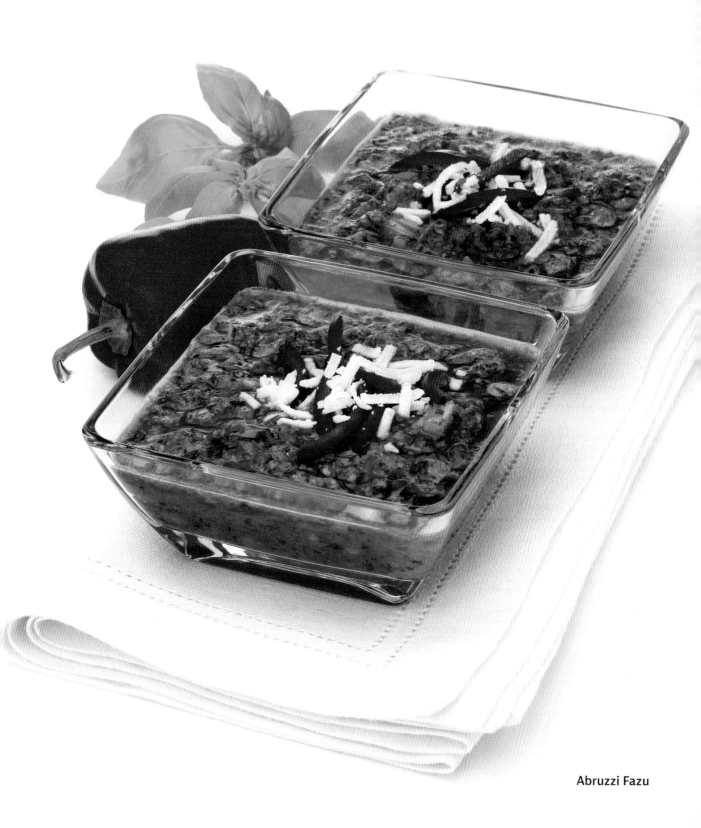

Abruzzi Fazu

Gazpacho A Go-Go

Calories	221
Fat	16 g
Sat fat	0
Protein	5 g
Carbohydrate	18 g
Fiber	4 g

Gazpacho soup is familiar to many, but this rendition makes a great luncheon smoothie. We increased the amounts so you could use this recipe to serve as a dinner soup later in the day, but the nutritional analysis is based on 1 serving. The ingredients blend to make a delicious beverage and an excellent nutrient and phytochemical profile. We didn't add salt, although a few of our tasters liked it better with a dash of sea salt.

	¼	peeled large cucumber (1¼ oz/65 g)
	4	medium plum (Roma) tomatoes (1 lb/490 g)
	½	seeded medium serrano chile (¼ oz/6 g)
	½	seeded ribbed large red bell pepper (3½ oz/100 g)
	¼	medium onion (2 oz/58 g)
	1 slice (½ inch/1 cm)	crusty whole-grain bread (1¼ oz/36 g)
	1	clove garlic
	2 tbsp (30 mL)	walnuts (1 oz/25 g)
	1 tbsp (15 mL)	red wine vinegar
	2 tbsp (30 mL)	olive oil

1. Wash all produce well.

2. Add all ingredients to blender and pulse (use the stop/start toggle switch several times) until desired consistency.

Makes 3 servings (3¼ cups/800 mL/810 g)

Phytochemicals

ALA, allicin, alpha- and beta-carotene, anthocyanin, caffeic acid, campesterol, capsaicin, chlorogenic acid, chlorophyll, cucurbitacin, diallyl sulfide, ellagic acid, eugenol, ferulic acid, glucosinolates, isorhamnetin, kaempferol, limonene, lycopene, myricetin, naringenin, oleanolic acid, phytoene, phytofluene, phytosterols, quercetin, rutin, saponin, squalene, zeaxanthin

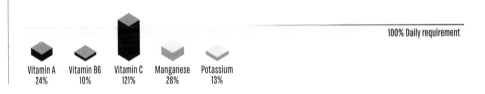

					100% Daily requirement
Vitamin A 24%	Vitamin B6 10%	Vitamin C 121%	Manganese 28%	Potassium 13%	

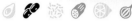

Beany Riced Avocado

You can drink this for a meal replacement or you can use this as a hot soup or a sauce for grains. Adding spices and herbs will add to the impressive phytochemical list, so you can experiment with the different flavors.

	½	peeled medium cucumber (3½ oz/100 g)
	½	peeled pitted large avocado (3½ oz/100 g)
	1 slice (1 inch/2.5 cm)	lemon (1½ oz/40 g)
	⅓ cup (75 mL)	black beans (3 oz/80 g)
	½	medium sweet onion (1 oz/25 g)
	¼ cup (60 mL)	cooked brown rice (2 oz/50 g)
	½ cup (125 mL)	water

1. Wash all produce well. Remove rind and seeds from lemon.

2. Add all ingredients to blender and process until desired consistency, adding more liquid if the mixture is too thick.

Makes 2 servings (2 cups/500 mL/515 g)

Calories	167
Fat	7 g
Sat fat	1 g
Protein	5 g
Carbohydrate	24 g
Fiber	8 g

Super Enhancer Tip

Try any of the high-antioxidant spices and herbs for a flavor and phytochemical boost. Cumin, turmeric and oregano would work well with the other ingredients.

100% Daily requirement

Vitamin C 29%   Folate 10%   Vitamin K 13%   No minerals present at 10% level

Phytochemicals
ALA, anthocyanin, beta-sitosterol, caffeic acid, chlorogenic acid, cryptoxanthin, cucurbitacin, ferulic acid, glucosinolates, isorhamnetin, kaempferol, lutein, oleanolic acid, oleic acid, phytosterols, quercetin, rutin, saponin, squalene, tartaric acid

Curried Avocado Dal

Calories	125
Fat	8 g
Sat fat	1 g
Protein	4 g
Carbohydrate	12 g
Fiber	7 g

Super Enhancer Tip

Add 2 tbsp (30 mL) ground flaxseed to increase protein, fiber, phytochemicals and omega-3 fats.

Here's a recipe with a twist on the avocado from the continent of India, where legumes such as lentils are called dal. This makes a wonderful lunch beverage, and you can boost the protein with flax. Heat it up and enjoy with a crusty piece of whole-grain bread and a slice of aged cheese for a light and quick dinner.

	½	peeled medium cucumber (3½ oz/100 g)
	½	peeled pitted large avocado (3½ oz/100 g)
	1 slice (1 inch/2.5 cm)	lemon (1½ oz/40 g)
	3 tbsp (45 mL)	canned or cooked lentils (1½ oz/38 g)
	¼	medium sweet onion (1 oz/25 g)
	1	clove garlic
	½ tsp (2 mL)	curry powder
	½ cup (125 mL)	water

1. Wash all produce well; remove rind and seeds from lemon.

2. Add all ingredients to blender and process until desired consistency, adding more liquid if the mixture is too thick.

Makes 2 servings (2 cups/500 mL/470 g)

Phytochemicals

ALA, allicin, anthocyanin, beta-sitosterol, caffeic acid, chlorogenic acid, cinnamic acid, cryptoxanthin, cucurbitacin, curcumin, diallyl sulfide, eugenol, ferulic acid, glucosinolates, isorhamnetin, kaempferol, limonene, lutein, luteolin, oleanolic acid, oleic acid, phytosterols, quercetin, rutin, saponin, squalene, tartaric acid

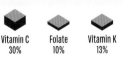

100% Daily requirement

Vitamin C 30% Folate 10% Vitamin K 13% No minerals present at 10% level

Curried Avocado Dal

Pepper Hummus Smoothie

Calories	155
Fat	2 g
Sat fat	0
Protein	9 g
Carbohydrate	25 g
Fiber	2 g

Super Enhancer Tip

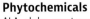 Stir in 2 tbsp (30 mL) ground flaxseed to add 4 grams of fiber, additional protein and phytochemicals and omega-3 fatty acids.

This savory beverage brings the flavors of red pepper hummus. It's great as a meal replacement to drink on the run, or heat it up and enjoy with a toasted whole wheat pita.

	½	seeded ribbed large red bell pepper (3½ oz/100 g)
	½ cup (125 mL)	chickpeas (3 oz/80 g)
	2 tbsp (30 mL)	nonfat Greek yogurt (2 oz/55 g)
	1 tbsp (15 mL)	sesame seeds (¼ oz/9 g)
	¼ tsp (1 mL)	ground turmeric
	½ tsp (2 mL)	ground cumin
	2 tbsp (30 mL)	water

1. Wash all produce well.

2. Add all ingredients to blender and process until desired consistency.

Makes 1 serving (1 cup/250 mL/270 g)

Phytochemicals

ALA, alpha-carotene, caffeic acid, campesterol, capsaicin, chlorogenic acid, cinnamic acid, cryptoxanthin, curcumin, eugenol, hesperidin, limonene, lutein, luteolin, phytoene, phytofluene, phytosterols, quercetin, zeaxanthin

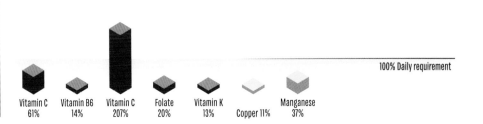

100% Daily requirement

Vitamin C 61% | Vitamin B6 14% | Vitamin C 207% | Folate 20% | Vitamin K 13% | Copper 11% | Manganese 37%

Samurai Smoothie

Tamari sauce is the Japanese version of soy sauce, and many people describe it as having a more mellow and deep flavor. You can easily substitute soy sauce, though, and both are rich sources of antioxidants, although they are high in sodium. You can either sip this as a savory beverage or enjoy with Japanese rice or soba noodles.

	2	stalks asparagus (½ oz/18 g)
	¼ cup (60 mL)	seeded ribbed red bell pepper (1 oz/30 g)
	1 piece (½ inch/1 cm)	gingerroot (⅛ oz/3g)
	¼ cup (60 mL)	wheatgrass (⅛ oz/4 g)
	¼ cup (60 mL)	silken tofu (1½ oz/40 g)
	2 tbsp (30 mL)	water
	1 tsp (5 mL)	tamari or soy sauce

1. Wash all produce well. Break off lower portion of asparagus stalks and peel ginger.

2. Add asparagus, red pepper, ginger, wheatgrass, tofu and water to blender and process until desired consistency.

3. Stir in tamari sauce.

Makes 1 serving (1 cup/250 mL/290 g)

Calories	40
Fat	1 g
Sat fat	0
Protein	4 g
Carbohydrate	4 g
Fiber	1 g

Super Enhancer Tip

This super-low-calorie beverage or soup can be enhanced with ground flaxseed, which will double the fiber and boost the protein, too.

Phytochemicals
ALA, alpha- and beta-carotene, caffeic acid, campesterol, capsaicin, chlorogenic acid, chlorophyll, cinnamic acid, cryptoxanthin, diosgenin, eugenol, hesperidin, inositol, isoflavones, lignans, limonene, lutein, oleic acid, phenols, phytoene, phytofluene, phytosterols, quercetin, zeaxanthin

100% Daily requirement

Vitamin A 21%   Vitamin C 65%   Vitamin K 11%   No minerals present at 10% level

Szechuan Smoothie

Calories	75
Fat	0
Sat fat	0
Protein	6 g
Carbohydrate	10 g
Fiber	4 g

The soy sauce and tofu provide an Asian touch to this savory beverage. It can be heated and served with rice or noodles for dinner. As a soup, try whisking in chopped green onion and water chestnuts.

⅓	seeded ribbed large red bell pepper (1 oz/32 g)
2 tbsp (30 mL)	silken tofu (1 oz/30 g)
¼ cup (60 mL)	water
1 piece (½ inch/1 cm)	gingerroot (⅛ oz/3g)
1 cup (250 mL)	chopped cabbage (2¼ oz/65 g)
1 tsp (5 mL)	dark soy sauce

1. Wash all produce well and peel ginger.

2. Add pepper, tofu, water and ginger to blender and process.

3. Add cabbage and soy sauce and process until desired consistency.

Makes 1 serving (¾ cup/175 mL/195 g)

Phytochemicals
ALA, alpha carotene, caffeic acid, campesterol, capsaicin, chlorogenic acid, cinnamic acid, cryptoxanthin, cyanidins, eugenol, ferulic acid, gingerol, 6-dehydrogingerdione (DGE), hesperidin, isoflavones, indole-3-carbinol, kaempferol, lignans, limonene, lutein, lycopene, phytoene, phytofluene, phytosterols, quercetin, shogaols, sinigrin, zeaxanthin

Vitamin A 23%	Vitamin B6 11%	Vitamin C 160%	Vitamin B6 14%	Folate 20%	Magnesium 10%	Manganese 12%	Molybdenum 11%	Potassium 14%

100% Daily requirement

Szechuan Smoothie

Beany Zucchini

Calories	101
Fat	1 g
Sat fat	0
Protein	6 g
Carbohydrate	19 g
Fiber	5 g

The only vegetable missing in this takeoff on ratatouille is eggplant. While we love eggplant, it doesn't work too well as a raw ingredient. But if you're adventurous, give that a try, too.

This is the perfect savory beverage in the summer, because many of these ingredients are garden favorites. Try it heated as a rich and satisfying soup accompanied by crusty multigrain bread, an exotic cheese and a glass of red wine.

	1	small baby zucchini (3½ oz/100 g)
	1	medium tomato (7 oz/200 g)
	½	seeded ribbed large red bell pepper (3 oz/90 g)
	¼	medium sweet onion (2 oz/60 g)
	½ cup (125 mL)	cannellini or other white beans (3 oz/90 g)
	1	clove garlic
	¼ cup (60 mL)	fresh basil leaves (¼ oz/6 g)
	¼ cup (60 mL)	water

1. Wash all produce well. Cut ends off zucchini.

2. Add all ingredients to blender and process, adding more liquid if needed to reach desired consistency.

Makes 2 servings (2½ cups/625 mL/625 g)

Phytochemicals
ALA, allicin, alpha carotene, anthocyanin, caffeic acid, campesterol, capsaicin, chlorogenic acid, chlorophyll, cinnamic acid, cryptoxanthin, cucurbitacin, diallyl sulfide, eugenol, ferulic acid, geraniol, glucosinolates, hesperidin, isoflavones, isorhamnetin, kaempferol, lignans, limonene, lutein, lycopene, naringenin, oleanolic acid, phytoene, phytofluene, phytosterols, quercetin, rutin, saponin, secoisolariciresinol, squalene, zeaxanthin

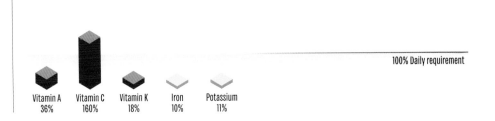

100% Daily requirement

Vitamin A	Vitamin C	Vitamin K	Iron	Potassium
36%	160%	18%	10%	11%

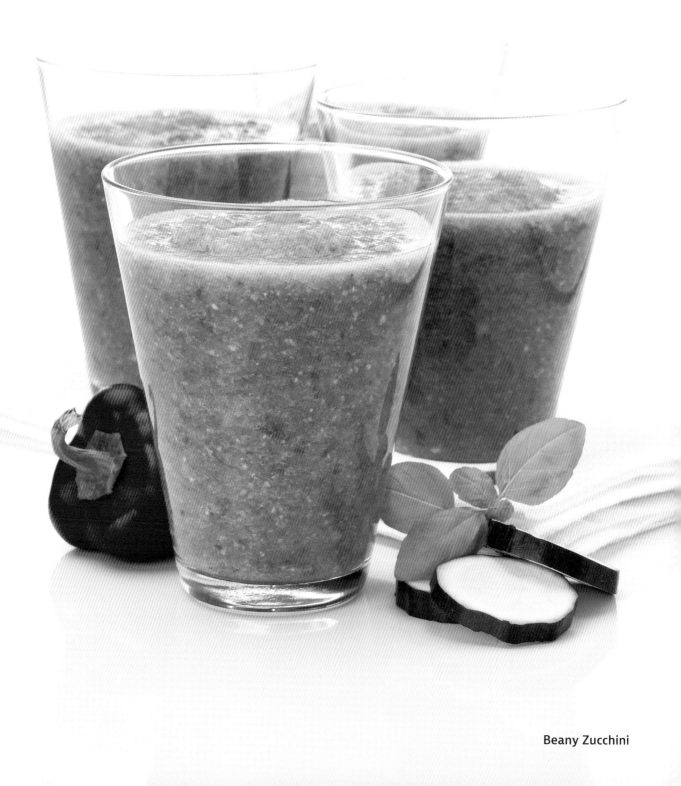

Beany Zucchini

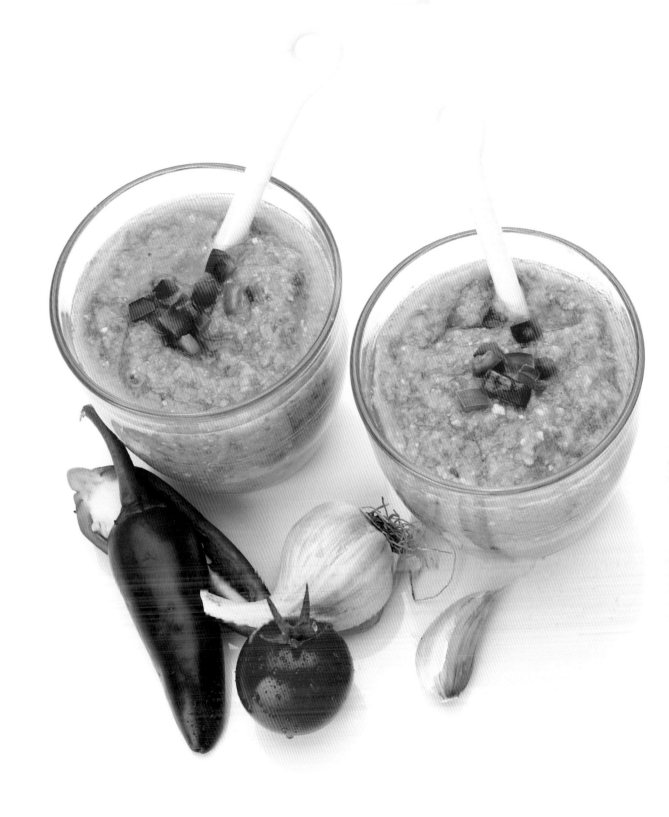

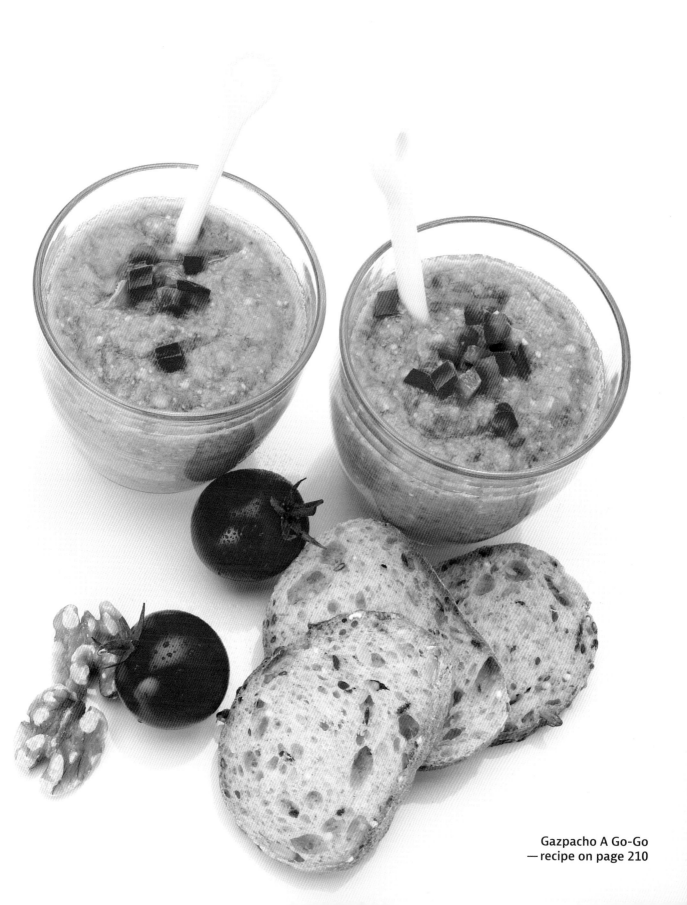

Gazpacho A Go-Go
— recipe on page 210

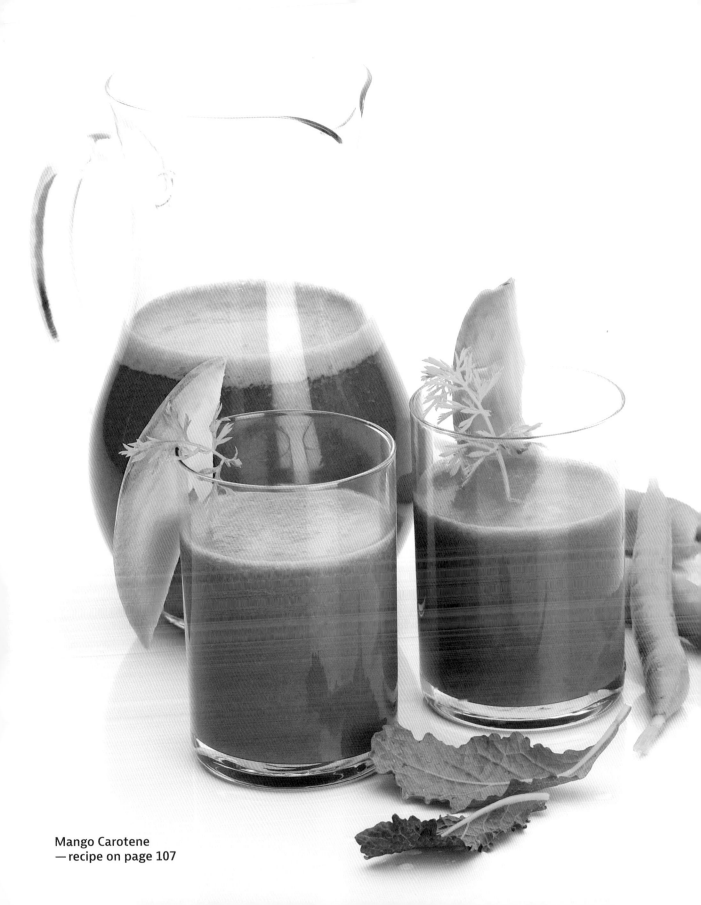

Mango Carotene
— recipe on page 107

Glossary

Allicin, Alliin, Allyl cysteine, Allyl disulfide
Phytochemicals in garlic with high antioxidant activity. Studies have shown these compounds have antimicrobial, anticancer, anti-inflammatory and anticlotting effects. In addition, they may lower blood cholesterol levels. When garlic is crushed, the enzyme alliinase breaks down alliin to form allicin, which also breaks down to form other compounds. The enzyme is inactivated by cooking, so food scientists recommend crushing or chopping garlic and allowing it to stand for about 10 minutes before cooking.

Alpha-linolenic acid (ALA) An essential nutrient that is a form of omega-3 fatty acid found in plants. Sources include walnuts and the oils from canola, soybeans, flaxseed/linseed and olives. A small amount can be converted to two other omega-3 fatty acids, docosahexaenoic acid (DHA) and eicosapentaenoic acid (EPA) — the oils in fish — which may reduce the risk of cardiovascular disease and diseases involving inflammation.

Anacardic acid An acid compound with antimicrobial effects and possible anticancer activity. Sources include mangos and cashews.

Anthocyanins Flavonoid compounds that provide purple and red pigment to fruits and vegetables. They act as antioxidants and may protect against cardiovascular disease and cancer. Sources include blueberries, cranberries, blackberries, black currants, red currants, cherries and purple grapes.

Anthocyanidins A large group of flavonoid compounds, one of which is cyanidin, consisting of blue and red pigments. Studies indicate that the compounds have anticancer properties. Sources include berries, red and blue grapes and red wine.

Anticlotting, Anticoagulant Compound that prevents clotting of the blood. The formation of a blood clot is an important step in the development of cardiovascular disease.

Antimicrobials Substances that prevent the growth of microorganisms. Antimicrobials include a wide-ranging group of additives and naturally occurring compounds that protect food from spoilage that results in food poisoning by inactivating microbes such as bacteria, yeasts, molds and other fungi.

Antioxidant Compounds that prevent oxidative damage by becoming oxidized themselves. Oxidative damage is the underlying cause of cardiovascular disease, cancer, diabetes and other diseases and conditions. Essential nutrients that act as antioxidants include vitamins C and E and selenium. Many phytochemicals, such as carotenoids and polyphenols, act as antioxidants.

Apigenin A flavonoid of the flavone subgroup that may have anticancer effects. Sources include parsley, thyme, celery and hot (chile) peppers.

Apoptosis Programmed cell death, or cell suicide, which is important in many natural processes and in the prevention of cancer.

Bergapten A phytochemical with anti-inflammatory, anticancer and anticlotting effects. Sources include carrots and essential oils from bergamot orange and other citrus fruits.

Beta-carotene (*also see* Carotenoids) A yellow-orange pigment in the carotenoid family, found in many fruits and vegetables. It functions as an antioxidant, and it is a precursor to retinol, the active form of vitamin A in the body. Sources include carrots, apricots, cantaloupe, broccoli and dark leafy greens (the orange pigment is present in dark leafy greens and other green veggies but is masked by the chlorophyll).

Beta-glucans Compounds in the cell wall of plants, fungi, bacteria and yeast. They may enhance the immune function, lower levels of cholesterol and help prevent cancer. Sources include some mushrooms, grain brans and seaweed.

Betaine A phytochemical that may have cardio-protective effects. Sources include beets, spinach, fish and baked goods.

Beta-sitosterol (*also see* Phytosterols) A plant sterol with antioxidant and antidiabetes activity. It also lowers blood levels of cholesterol. Dietary sources include nuts, seeds, berries, wheat germ, bran from various grains, soybeans and some vegetable oils.

Betulinic acid A compound found in rosemary and the bark from several tree species, has antimicrobial, anticancer and anti-inflammatory effects.

Caffeic acid A compound in the hydroxycinnamic acid group. Studies have shown it to have antioxidant, anti-inflammatory and anticancer effects. Sources include apples, artichokes, basil, oregano, pear and thyme.

Calorie (or kilocalorie) A unit of measure of energy from food, which can also be expressed as kilojoules, with 1 calorie equaling 4.184 kilojoules. Most adult require 1500 to 2800 calories a day, depending on age, gender and physical activity level.

Campesterol (*see* Phytosterols) Camphene A phytochemical with antioxidant and blood-cholesterol-lowering effects. Sources include parsnips, rosemary and celery leaf.

Capsaicin A phytochemical in hot peppers (chiles) that produces a burning sensation. Research shows it has numerous biologic effects, including analgesic, anti-inflammatory, anticancer and antioxidant.

Carbohydrate A group of essential nutrients that serve as the major energy source for the body, providing 4 calories (16.7 kJ) per gram. Carbohydrate includes starches, sugars and fiber. Simple carbohydrates, or sugars, include those naturally occurring in fruit (fructose) and milk (lactose). So-called "added sugars" are those used as ingredients in commercial products such as soft drinks, candy and desserts. In addition to causing dental caries, sugar contributes no nutrients but significant calories, which can lead to a low-nutrient-dense diet and weight gain. Health agencies recommend no more than 100 and 150 calories from added sugar per day for women and men, respectively.

Cardiovascular disease (CVD) A group of diseases affecting the heart and/or blood vessels, with the major forms consisting of myocardial infarction (heart attack), stroke and high blood pressure. It is the leading cause of death in most industrialized countries. The underlying processes include inflammation and oxidative damage.

Carnosic acid, Carnosol A phytochemical in sage and rosemary; some studies show it may have antimicrobial, antioxidant and other anticancer effects.

Carotenoids A family of pigments comprising two main groups, carotenes and xanthophylls, and consisting of over 600 individual compounds found in plants. The human body can convert 50 of these compounds to active vitamin A. Many carotenoids are antioxidants that vary in potency, and they also stimulate immune function and inhibit cell proliferation that is linked to cancer. The five main carotenoids include alpha-carotene, beta-carotene, lutein, cryptoxanthin and lycopene.

Catechins, Catechol Antioxidant flavanol compounds, and the related compound epicatechin, found in cocoa beans. Catechol is another compound with similarities but is also used as the class name for catechins.

Chlorogenic acid, Neochlorogenic acid
A cinnamic acid with antioxidant, anticancer, antihypertensive and antidiabetes effects. It has recently been studied as a weight loss agent, and it may also be one of the active ingredients that act as a laxative in prunes. Neochlorogenic acid is a chemical isomer of chlorogenic acid. Sources include sour cherries, peaches, prunes and coffee bean extract.

Chlorophyll Green pigment in plants, involved in photosynthesis. Research shows it blocks carcinogens from initiating cancer development. Sources include green vegetables, sea vegetables and leafy green vegetables.

Cholesterol A lipid that is an important constituent of cell membranes and for some hormones. It is made by the liver and also found in animal foods. Cholesterol circulates in the blood via carriers called lipoproteins, which include high-density lipoprotein (HDL) and low-density lipoprotein (LDL). HDL ("good cholesterol") carries cholesterol away from arteries and to the liver for removal and protects against heart attacks. High levels of LDL ("bad cholesterol") increase risk of heart attack.

Cinnamic acid, Hydroxycinnamic acid (a derivative) Polyphenols (and several specific derivatives) with antioxidant and antimicrobial activity. Sources of various derivatives include cinnamon, coffee, artichokes, strawberries, apples, pears and pineapples.

Coumarins A family of compounds, found in plants and microorganisms, with many biologic activities that include anticlotting, anti-inflammatory, anticancer, antidiuretic, antimicrobial and antioxidant effects. Sources include carrots, celery, cinnamon, cocoa, corn, dates, sour cherries and tarragon.

Coumestrol A phytoestrogen in the coumestans family. Limited studies have reported anticancer and anti-inflammatory effects, particularly in lung tissue. Sources include soybeans and other legumes, alfalfa, spinach and Brussels sprouts.

Cruciferous vegetables Vegetables containing sulfur, such as broccoli, cauliflower, kale and Brussels sprouts. They contain phytochemicals known as indoles, as well as dithiolthiones, which have anticancer effects.

Cucurbitacin A group of phytochemicals with anticancer and anti-inflammatory effects. Sources include cucumbers and melons.

Cyanidin (*see* Anthocyanidin) Cryptoxanthin A carotenoid in fruits and vegetables that the body can convert to active vitamin A. It is also an antioxidant.

Daidzein An isoflavone found in soybeans and other legumes and alfalfa sprouts. Studies have shown anticancer and bone protective effects.

% Daily Value A reference standard used on food labels in North America that describes a food's content of specific nutrients and constituents compared to the Dietary Reference Intakes and daily reference values.

Diabetes mellitus A chronic disease caused either by a lack of insulin or inadequate response to insulin, resulting in elevated blood glucose levels. Type 1 diabetes typically develops in childhood or adolescence, while type 2 diabetes usually develops in adulthood. Type 2 diabetes is often associated with obesity, particularly excess abdominal fat. Diabetes increases the risk for cardiovascular disease, amputations, blindness and kidney disease.

Dietary Reference Intakes (DRI) A set of nutrient intake recommendations established by the US Institute of Medicine and currently used by the United States and Canada. The DRIs include four nutrient levels: Estimated Average Requirements (EAR), Recommended Dietary Allowances (RDA), Adequate Intake (AI), and Tolerable Upper Intake Levels. Of these, only the RDA and AI represent recommended levels of intake, and the recommendation is based on age and gender.

Diosgenin A phytochemical with anti-inflammatory and cholesterol-lowering effects. Sources include asparagus, carrot and bitter melon.

Diosmin A flavonoid related to hesperidin, with anticancer, antioxidant, blood-glucose-lowering and anti-inflammatory effects. Sources include lemons and rosemary.

Ellagic acid An antioxidant compound in the phenolic acid group. Some studies indicate it may lower blood pressure. Sources include grapes, walnuts, pomegranate, strawberries, grapes, cranberries and blackberries.

Eugenol A phytochemical with antimicrobial, antioxidant, anticancer and anti-inflammatory effects. Sources include blueberries, bay leaves, basil, cinnamon, cloves and turmeric.

Fats, Fatty acids An essential nutrient that is chemically a lipid. Triglyceride is the form of fat in foods and the fat stored in the body. In foods, fat provides 9 calories per gram, more than twice the amount from carbohydrate or protein, which both provide 4 calories per gram. Triglyceride contains fatty acids, and the presence of double bonds between carbon atoms identifies the fat as unsaturated, or no double bonds, as a saturated fat. A high dietary intake of saturated fat can raise blood cholesterol in some people, and a high intake of unsaturated fat may improve blood cholesterol levels.

Ferulic acid An acid in the hydroxycinnamic group that functions as an antioxidant. Sources include oats, artichoke, orange, rice, pineapple, peanut and apple.

Fiber Compounds in plants that humans do not have digestive enzymes to degrade. The two types are insoluble and soluble fiber. Insoluble fiber, which includes cellulose, hemicellulose and lignin, helps in waste elimination. Sources include wheat bran, whole-grain breads and cereals and vegetables. Soluble fiber, which includes pectins, gums and mucilages, may reduce levels of glucose and cholesterol in the blood. Sources include fruits, legumes, oats and barley. Both types can be degraded by bacteria colonizing the large intestine, and they are considered prebiotics in that they promote bacterial growth.

Fish oil (see Omega-3 fatty acid)

Flavonoids Plant-based compounds high in fruits, vegetables, nuts, tea and coffee. These compounds include flavanols (which includes catechins), flavones, flavonols, flavanones, isoflavones and anthocyanins. They can act as antioxidants, anti-inflammatory and anticancer agents.

Flavonols Flavonoid compounds, which include kaempferol, myricetin and quercetin. Flavonols are antioxidants and also help regulate blood flow and blood pressure.

Free radicals (*see* Reactive oxygen species)

Friedelin A phytochemical in pears with anti-inflammatory and diuretic (promoting urination) effects.

Gallic acid A phenolic acid compound with anti-microbial and antioxidant activity. Sources include mango, blackberries, raspberries, tea and soy foods.

Genistein An isoflavone found in plant foods, especially soy. Studies suggest that genistein may protect against heart disease by reducing blood cholesterol level and inhibiting blood clotting.

Geraniol A phytochemical with anti-inflammatory, anticancer and antimicrobial effects. Sources include basil, carrots, rosemary, tea and thyme.

Glucosinolates Sulfur compounds in cruciferous vegetables that break down to form many different types of isothiocyanates. These compounds have several important health effects, which vary depending on the compound from the specific vegetable. The main effect studied is protection against cancer.

Glycemic index (GI) A measure of the extent to which a carbohydrate-containing food raises blood glucose and insulin in comparison to a reference food, which is usually white bread. Foods high in fiber and fat typically have a lower GI. Studies suggest that a high GI diet can promote obesity and increase the risk for type 2 diabetes. People with diabetes may have better control of blood glucose levels (glycemic control) by consuming a diet that is predominantly based on low GI foods. Carbohydrate foods with a low GI include legumes, most vegetables, many fruits and whole-grain breads and cereals.

Glycemic load (GL) A ranking system for foods based on the glycemic index (GI). Most foods will have a similar GI and GL, although some exceptions occur. The GL can be determined by calculating: GI x (the amount of carbohydrate in grams per serving) ÷ 100.

Glycetin An isoflavone that studies show has antioxidant, anticancer and bone protective effects. Sources include soybeans and other legumes.

Goitrogens Compounds naturally occurring in plant foods; interfere with the production of the thyroid hormones. Goitrogens are present in peanut skins, cabbage, cauliflower and turnips, but cooking destroys them. Goitrogens could potentially cause goiter, but this is unlikely.

Hesperetin A flavanone with antimicrobial and anticancer effects. Sources include grapefruit and mint.

Hesperidin A flavanone compound, along with the related compound neohesperidin, in citrus fruits; has powerful antioxidant activity and may also have other anticancer effects.

Indoles, indole-3-carbinol Phytochemical group that includes indole-3-carbinol, a compound with antioxidant, anticancer and anti-inflammatory effects. Sources include cruciferous vegetables and rutabaga.

Inositol A compound similar to glucose, found in many plants and animals. In plants, it is present at phytic acid (see Phytic acid). Although it is not considered an essential nutrient, new research suggests that problems in the body's metabolism of the compound may be related to diseases such as diabetes and multiple sclerosis.

Insulin A hormone produced by the pancreas; regulates metabolism of carbohydrates, lipids and proteins to maintain blood sugar levels within a healthy range.When its production is inadequate, or if insulin is ineffective, the result is diabetes mellitus.

Inulin A phytochemical with anticancer, immune-enhancing and blood-glucose- and cholesterol-lowering effects. It is also an excellent probiotic, serving as a food source for bacteria living in the colon. Sources include asparagus, garlic, leeks, onions, banana and wheat.

Isoflavones A type of phytoestrogen found in plant foods, especially in soy products (see Phytoestrogens, Genistein).

Isorhamnetin A flavonol with antioxidant activity. Sources include broccoli, apples, berries and grapefruit.

Isoquercetin (*see* Quercetin)

Isothiocyanates Plant compounds that contain sulfur and are formed from the breakdown of glucosinolates. They have several beneficial effects on health, including anticancer and blood-cholesterol-lowering effects and reduction in blood clotting, important aspects in the prevention of cardiovascular disease.

Kaempferol A flavonoid with numerous biologic effects, which include anticancer, antimicrobial, anti-inflammatory and antioxidant effects. Sources include strawberries, cruciferous vegetables, beans, peas and spinach.

Lignans Plant-based compounds with antioxidant activity and that block estrogen activity in cells. May protect against breast and ovarian cancers, heart disease and osteoporosis.

Liminoids A group of compounds — which includes limonin, limonene, limonexic acid and several important flavonoids — in citrus fruits and other plants.. Studies indicate these compounds have varied effects, including antiviral and anticancer.

Lipids Compounds that include triglyceride, phospholipids and sterols. Triglyceride is the form of fat in foods and stored in the body. Phospholipids are important in the formation of cell membrane. Sterols include cholesterol, steroid hormones and phytosterols in plants.

Lipoic acid (LA, Thioctic acid, also known as Alpha-lipoic acid) A sulfur-containing acid with antioxidant activity that is essential for many animals but not humans, since the body can synthesize the compound. It is found in some plant foods, and studies have suggested potential benefits related to cardiovascular disease, cancer and Alzheimer's disease.

Lupeol A phytochemical with antioxidant, anticancer, anti-inflammatory and blood-glucose-and blood-pressure-lowering effects. Sources include carrots and the seeds of many plants.

Lutein A carotenoid, in the subclass xanthophyll, that exists as an isomer as zeaxanthin;, both are potent antioxidants. Lutein is found in the retina of the eye and zeaxanthin is contained in the macula. Some studies suggest it may be helpful in preventing cataracts and macular degeneration.

Luteolin A flavonoid compound that has antioxidant, anticancer, anti-inflammatory and immune- enhancing effects. Sources include green bell peppers, thyme, oregano, carrots, olive oil, rosemary and oranges.

Lycopene A carotenoid with no vitamin A activity but with high antioxidant capacity. Research points to a role in the prevention of cancers, particularly prostate cancer. Sources include tomatoes, red bell peppers, watermelons and papaya.

Matairesinol A lignan compound that occurs in foods with the related compound secoisolariciresinol. It may protect against cardiovascular disease and cancer. Sources include strawberries, carrots, flaxseed, sesame seeds and broccoli.

Mangiferin A compound in mangos with antimicrobial and antioxidant effects.

Minerals Inorganic elements present in foods in a basic form.

Monounsaturated fats Dietary fats (see Fats) that have one double bond between adjacent carbon atoms on a fatty acid and are therefore unsaturated. Research has shown beneficial effects in protecting against cardiovascular disease. The effects include lowering levels of cholesterol in the blood and reducing inflammation. Some food sources, such as olive oil, contain antioxidant phytochemicals that may also help prevent cancer. Monounsaturated fats include olive oil, canola oil, peanut oil and sesame oil; food sources include avocados and many nuts and seeds.

Myricetin (*see* Flavonol)

Naringenin A flavanone with antimicrobial, antioxidant, anticancer and anti-inflammatory effects. Sources include grapefruit, oranges, oregano, sour cherries, tarragon and thyme.

Neohesperidin (*see* Hesperidin)

Nutrients Compounds needed for specific body functions and are necessary for life. Some nutrients can be made by the body, but those which cannot must be obtained through the diet and are called essential nutrients. The six classes of essential nutrients are carbohydrates, protein, fats, vitamins, minerals and water.

Nutrient density A measure of the nutrients in a food in relation to the energy, in calories, it contains. Nutrient-dense foods are those high in essential nutrients and health-promoting phytochemicals and low in calories. Currently, there is not an established standard for nutrient density.

Oleanolic acid A compound in garlic and other plants; may protect against viruses and cancer.

Oleic acid A phytochemical with anti-inflammatory, anticancer and blood-cholesterol-lowering effects. Sources include avocados, olives and many nuts and seeds.

Omega-3 fats, fatty acids Polyunsaturated fatty acids contained in fish and also in some plants in the form of alpha-linolenic acid (ALA). In fish, the fatty acids are eicosapentaenoic (EPA) and docosahexaenoic acid (DHA). The body can convert ALA to EPA and DHA, but the rate is low, from 8% to 15%. These fats have many effects, especially anti-inflammatory, but they may also enhance immune function. Additional cardiovascular benefits include lowering of blood pressure and improvement in overall cardiovascular function.

Oxalic acid, Oxalate A compound present in many plant foods that interferes with calcium absorption. In the body, oxalic acid combines with magnesium and calcium and is excreted as oxalate. Oxalate is the basis for the most common type of kidney stones, and people with a history of these stones should avoid foods high in the compound, including rhubarb, beets, berries, spinach, endive, green beans, sweet potato, Swiss chard, collard greens, nuts, tea and chocolate.

Oxidative damage Damage to the body's compounds and tissues by the process of oxidation, in which a substance combines with oxygen and causes the loss of electrons. The oxidizing compounds are known as free radicals, one type of reactive oxygen species (ROS). They can arise from pollution, exposure to sunlight, cigarette smoke and oxidized compounds in foods. The body produces ROS as part of the immune response in normal metabolism and during intense exercise. Oxidative damage is involved in cardiovascular disease, cancer and other diseases.

Pelargonidin An anthocyanidin compound that is an antioxidant. Sources include red kidney beans, pomegranates, cranberries, berries and plums.

Phenols (Phenolic compounds) A large group of compounds in many plants; consists of several subgroups. Studies have shown that they possess important biologic effects, including antioxidant, anti-inflammatory and anticancer effects.

Phytic acid, Phytate A compound, found in plant seeds, grain husks and legumes, consisting of a ring of phosphorus groups. It has the ability to bind other compounds, including essential minerals, and prevent their absorption. It may also be beneficial to health because it has antioxidant activity, antidiabetic, cholesterol-lowering, and anticancer effects.

Phytochemical Also called phytonutrients. Any compound contained in plants that is not an essential nutrient, many of which may possess beneficial health effects.

Phytoene, Phytofluene Carotenoid compounds that are precursors to lycopene and that may also have biologic effects not yet known. Sources include oranges, watermelon, apricots, cantaloupe, pink grapefruit, pumpkin, mango, papaya, peaches, prunes and tomatoes.

Phytoestrogens Compounds in some plants with chemical structures and functions similar to estrogen. Some key phytoestrogens are isoflavones and flavones. Studies show a potential reduction in breast and prostate cancers and cardiovascular disease. Food sources include nuts, seeds and soy products.

Phytosterols Plant-based compounds, one of which is campesterol, that are similar to human cholesterol. Sterol esters and stanol esters are two groups that lower blood cholesterol by blocking absorption of cholesterol from foods. Phytosterols are currently being added to margarine products and sold as supplements.

Piceatannol A compound in the stilbenoid family found in grapes. Studies have shown that it blocks certain viruses, and it also has metabolic effects related to insulin and fat tissue that may be beneficial.

Polyphenols A large and diverse group of compounds found in almost all plants. The compounds consist of several subgroups, distinguished by the two main groups, flavonoid and nonflavonoid. Polyphenols have a wide range of potential beneficial functions in the body and appear to protect against chronic diseases.

Probiotics, Prebiotics A probiotic is a food or supplement that contains live bacterial cultures thought to be beneficial for health. A prebiotic is a compound that serves as a food source for bacteria inhabiting the large intestine of humans and promotes their growth. Depending on the specific bacteria, prebiotics may promote either health or disease.

Procyanidin A flavonoid group that includes proanthocyanidins and possess antioxidant and anti-clotting activity.

Protein Essential nutrients containing nitrogen that provide energy (4 calories per gram). They are composed of amino acids, nine of which must be consumed through the diet. Proteins function as enzymes, antibodies and hormones, as well as key structural components of most body tissues.

Pterostilbene A compound in the stilbenoid group that is related to resveratrol. It exhibits antiviral, antidiabetic, anticancer, and cholesterol- and blood-pressure-lowering properties. It is found in grapes and blueberries.

Psyllium A seed from certain plant species containing a high amount of soluble fiber. It lowers blood cholesterol and helps regulate blood glucose level. Psyllium is added to commercial food products to increase fiber content and is used in laxative preparations.

Punicalagins A group of compounds that act as antioxidants. Pomegranates are a good source.

Quercetin, Isoquercetin Flavonols with antioxidant, anti-inflammatory and anticancer effects. Quercetin is most likely the compound responsible for grapefruit's ability to enhance the absorption of drugs in the stomach. Studies have shown a protective effect against ulcers and stomach cancers. Good sources include apples, onions, tea, asparagus, grapefruit and other citrus fruits.

Reactive oxygen species (ROS) Compounds with an unpaired electron that as a consequence cause oxidative damage to the body's structures and compounds, such as cell membranes, enzymes, DNA and LDL cholesterol. This damage is linked to many chronic diseases and conditions.

Resveratrol An anthocyanin compound found in the skins of red or black grapes and is a potent antioxidant. Researchers believe that the high level in red wine is one of the reasons for the lower rate of cardiovascular mortality among moderate consumers of red wine. More recent research links it to potentially slowing the aging process.

Rosmarinic acid, Rosmaridiphenol, Rosmanol Compounds found in rosemary and other plants; have antimicrobial, antioxidant and anti-inflammatory effects.

Rutin A compound in several plants; has antioxidant, antimicrobial, anticlotting and anti-inflammatory effects. Sources include citrus, buckwheat, apricots, tea, parsley and tomatoes.

Saponins Compounds found in some grains, nuts, grapes and legumes, such as soybeans. When shaken in a water solution, they foam, which is derivation of the name. In some foods, saponins may add a bitter taste. They act as antioxidants and anti-inflammatory agents and may protect against cancer. In addition, they appear to lower blood cholesterol levels. However, they may also reduce absorption of fat-soluble vitamins.

Secoisolariciresinol (see Matairesinol)

Shogaols Compounds derived from gingerols in gingerroot. They have been shown to have anticancer, antioxidant and anti-inflammatory effects.

Short-Chain Fatty Acids (SCFAs) Fatty acids (see Fats, Fatty acids) containing less than six carbons and with fewer calories than longer-chain fatty acids. Foods contain small amounts, and most SCFAs in the human body arise from bacteria digesting fiber in the colon. Soluble fiber is the best substrate for bacteria to make these fatty acids. Higher levels of SCFAs act as a laxative and cause diarrhea. Researchers are studying SCFAs for potential health benefits, especially in preventing colon cancer.

Squalene A phytochemical with antioxidant, antimicrobial, anticancer and immune-system-enhancing effects. Sources include cucumber, flaxseed, olives, sunflower seeds, sweet potatoes and tomatoes.

Sulforaphane An isothiocyanate found in cruciferous vegetables. It functions as an antioxidant and exhibits many effects that may protect against cancer. Studies have associated higher dietary intakes with lower rates of breast and prostate cancer, as well as lower blood pressure.

Tannins Polyphenols in many plant foods; cause an astringent, bitter taste. Condensed tannins are known as proanthocyanidins. The astringency is prized in red wines, but it also responsible for the undesirable taste of fruit that is not ripe. Tannins can block the absorption of essential minerals, especially iron and zinc, but may protect against cancer and cardiovascular disease through effects that include antioxidant, anticancer and anti-inflammatory. Sources include coffee, tea, nuts, berries and pomegranate.

Tartaric acid An antioxidant acid that is used as a food additive for this purpose. Sources include bananas, grapes, apricots, avocados and apples.

Theaflavins Polyphenol compounds that have antimicrobial, antioxidant and anticancer effects. Sources include coffee, cocoa and tea.

Tocopherols Fat-soluble compounds having vitamin E activity. Plant oils are good sources.

Triglycerides (see Fats)

Trigonelline A phytochemical with anti-inflammatory, anticancer, antimicrobial and blood-glucose- and cholesterol-lowering effects. Sources include green beans, coffee, peas and the seeds of many plants.

Umami The fifth human taste in addition to sweet, sour, salty and bitter. The word "umami" is Japanese, which translates as "delicious" and is described as imparting a meat-like flavor.

Ursolic acid Phytochemical with several anticancer effects and may protect the cardiovascular system. Sources include apples, basil, cranberries, rosemary, oregano and prunes

Vitamins Essential nutrients that regulate chemical reactions in the body. They must be obtained from the diet but are needed in minute quantities. A vitamin deficiency arises from an inadequate intake for a specific vitamin, which can be reversed by consuming it.

Whey The liquid that remains after the curd and cream are separated and removed from milk that has been coagulated to make products such as cheese. Nutritionally, it contains most of the lactose from the milk and some water-soluble nutrients. Whey protein can be isolated from the whey and is used as a nutritional supplement and as a food additive. Studies indicate that whey protein may be helpful in suppressing appetite and facilitating weight loss.

Zeaxanthin (see Lutein)

Useful Websites

Government Agencies

National Cancer Institute
www.cancer.gov
This site provides comprehensive information about cancer, including current research on the role of nutrition in prevention of the disease. Several free publications are available for download.

Centers for Disease Control and Prevention
www.cdc.gov
The CDC site contains content on diseases and covers many topics in the "Healthy Living" section. These topics include food safety, nutrition and disease prevention.

Food and Drug Administration, Consumer Publications
www.fda.gov
Topics on this site include dietary supplements, food recalls, basic nutrition and food labeling.

Office of Dietary Supplements, National Institutes of Health
http://ods.od.nih.gov
This is one of the best sites for accurate information on dietary supplements and naturally occurring phytochemicals. In addition to a searchable database, the site provides "Featured Dietary Supplement Fact Sheets" on specific supplements, many of which are essential nutrients.

National Center for Complementary and Alternative Medicine, National Institutes of Health
http://nccam.nih.gov
The NCCAM site covers topics related to complementary therapies that include dietary supplements. It now offers a series of fact sheets, available as an ebook, on herbs and botanicals.

Health Canada, the Canadian Nutrient File
www.hc-sc.gc.ca/fn-an/nutrition/fiche-nutri-data/index-eng.php
This Health Canada site offers a bilingual online nutrient database containing close to 6,000 foods. The main page has links to national nutrition and food policy reports, as well as nutrition education materials.

National Center for Biotechnology Information (PubMed)
www.ncbi.nlm.nih.gov
PubMed provides over 22 million citations for biomedical literature. While most of the research articles are available only as abstracts, full articles are available for many entries.

USDA Nutritional Analysis Database
http://ndb.nal.usda.gov
The USDA's nutritional analysis database is searchable for over 8,000 foods and also includes a section for international foods and one for phytochemicals.

Dietary Reference Intakes
http://fnic.nal.usda.gov/dietary-guidance/
dietary-reference-intakes
The DRI site contains the complete lists for nutrient intake recommendations. It also has links to dietary assessment tools, weight and obesity information, and nutrition assistance programs.

Non-government Agencies and Groups

Academy of Nutrition and Dietetics
www.eatright.org
Registered dietitians are the largest group of nutrition and dietetics professionals in the US. The site provides free consumer information on timely nutrition topics, including healthy weight, nutrition for different age groups, food allergies, and sports and exercise.

American Institute for Cancer Research
www.aicr.org/reduce-your-cancer-risk/diet/elements_phytochemicals.html
The AICR provides information on nutrition and cancer prevention with a specific section on phytochemicals. Consumers can also access healthy recipes organized by category.

American Diabetes Association
www.diabetes.org/home.jsp

American Heart Association
www.heart.org/HEARTORG

Cochrane Reviews
www.cochrane.org/cochrane-reviews
Provides systematic reviews of primary research in human health care and health policy.

Dietitians of Canada
www.dietitians.ca
This site represents Canada's dietitians and offers nutrition information for consumers. Some of the topics include food policy, nutrition for specific age groups and food regulation.

Fruit and Veggies More Matters
www.fruitsandveggiesmorematters.org
This site promotes fruit and vegetable consumption and offers a database of over 1,000 recipes. It also includes information on nutrition and disease prevention.

Linus Pauling Institute
http://lpi.oregonstate.edu
The Linus Pauling Institute is dedicated to preventing chronic disease and extending lifespan. The site provides videos on health and nutrition, as well as information on nutrients and phytochemicals.

National Soyfoods Directory
http://soyfoods.com
This site promotes the use of soyfoods by providing information on soy products, recipes and research. It contains a section, "What Doctors Are Saying About Soy and..." with topics that include prostate cancer, weight loss, menopause and glycemic index.

Nutrition Data
http://nutritiondata.self.com
A nutrient analysis database that provides analysis based on the DRIs.

Verified Health Quality
www.vhqfoods.ca/about-vhq.aspx
This site promotes the consumption of fruits and vegetables in Canada. It provides a search engine for fruits and vegetables that features nutrient analysis, as well as background information on what consumers should look for when selecting a particular item.

The World's Healthiest Foods
www.whfoods.com
This site is dedicated to improving consumer health through nutrition. It includes a database that provides the latest research on the nutrition and health attributes of numerous foods. It also offers recipes for many of the items in its database.

References

Blumenthal, Mark. *The ABC Clinical Guide to Herbs.* New York, NY: Thieme, 2003.

Carlson, MH, et al. The total antioxidant content of more than 3100 foods, beverages, spices, herbs and supplements used worldwide. Nutr J 2010;9:3.

Cheynier, V. Polyphenols in foods are more complex than often thought. Am J Clin Nutr 2005;81(suppl):223S–9S.

Divisi, D, et al. Diet and cancer. Acta Biomed 2006;77:118–123.

Dr. Duke's Phytochemical and Ethnobotanical Databases. Retrieved May 13, 2013, from www.ars-grin.gov/duke/plants.html.

Engelmann, NJ, Clinton, SK, Erdman, JW. Nutritional aspects of phytoene and phytofluene, carotenoid precursors to lycopene. Adv Nutr 2011;2: 51–61.

Fresco, P, et al. The anticancer properties of dietary polyphenols and its relation with apoptosis. Curr Pharm Design 2010;16:114–134.

Hyson, D. A comprehensive review of apples and apple components and their relationship to human health. Adv Nutr 2011;2:408–420.

Kennedy, DO, Wightman, EL. Herbal extracts and phytochemicals: Plant secondary metabolites and the enhancement of human brain function. Adv Nutr 2011;2:32–50.

Mahan, LK, Escott-Stump S, Raymond, JL. *Krause's Food & the Nutrition Care Process,* 13th ed. St. Louis, MO: Elsevier Health Sciences, 2011.

Manach, C, Scalbert, A, Morand, C, Rémésy, C, Jimenez, L. Polyphenols: Food sources and bioavailability. Am J Clin Nutr 2004;79:727–47.

Miller, PE, Snyder, DC. Phytochemicals and cancer risk: A review of the epidemiological evidence. Nutr Clin Pract 2012;27:599.

Pennington, JAT, Spungen, JS. *Bowes and Church's Food Values of Portions Commonly Used,* 19th ed. Baltimore, MD: Lippincott Williams & Wilkins, 2010.

Reinhard, Tonia. *Superfoods: The Healthiest Foods on the Planet*. Toronto, ON: Firefly Books, 2010.

Rolfes, SR, Pinna, K, Whitney, E. *Understanding Normal and Clinical Nutrition*. Belmont, CA: Wadsworth, 2011.

The Food Processor. Salem, OR: ESHA Research, 2012.

US Department of Agriculture, National Nutrient Database for Standard Reference, Release 25. Retrieved May 13, 2013, from www.ars.usda.gov/main/site_main.htm.

Wang, H, et al. The identification of antioxidants in dark soy sauce. Free Rad Res 2007; 41; 4:479–488.

Index